P9-CFP-331

# Basic
# Infection Control
## FOR HEALTH CARE
## PROVIDERS

SECOND EDITION

This book is dedicated to the love of my life—
my bride, Trisha.

# Basic
# Infection Control
# FOR HEALTH CARE PROVIDERS

## SECOND Edition

## Mike Kennamer, MPA, EMT-P
Director
Office of Workforce Development
Northeast Alabama Community College
Rainsville, Alabama

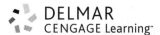

DELMAR
CENGAGE Learning™

Australia • Brazil • Japan • Korea • Mexico • Singapore • Spain • United Kingdom • United States

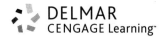

**Basic Infection Control for Health Care Providers, Second Edition**
Mike Kennamer

Vice President, Health Care Business Unit: William Brottmiller

Director of Learning Solutions: Matthew Kane

Managing Editor: Marah Bellegarde

Acquisitions Editor: Matthew Seeley

Marketing Director: Jennifer McAvey

Marketing Manager: Michele McTighe

Production Director: Carolyn Miller

Content Project Manager: Anne Sherman

© 2007 Delmar, Cengage Learning

ALL RIGHTS RESERVED. No part of this work covered by the copyright herein may be reproduced, transmitted, stored or used in any form or by any means graphic, electronic, or mechanical, including but not limited to photocopying, recording, scanning, digitizing, taping, Web distribution, information networks, or information storage and retrieval systems, except as permitted under Section 107 or 108 of the 1976 United States Copyright Act, without the prior written permission of the publisher.

For product information and technology assistance, contact us at
**Cengage Learning Customer & Sales Support, 1-800-354-9706**

For permission to use material from this text or product, submit all requests online at **www.cengage.com/permissions**
Further permissions questions can be emailed to **permissionrequest@cengage.com**

Library of Congress Control Number: 2006014983

ISBN-13: 978-1-4180-1978-5

ISBN-10: 1-4180-1978-X

**Delmar**
Executive Woods
5 Maxwell Drive
Clifton Park, NY 12065
USA

Cengage Learning is a leading provider of customized learning solutions with office locations around the globe, including Singapore, the United Kingdom, Australia, Mexico, Brazil, and Japan. Locate your local office at **international.cengage.com/region**

Cengage Learning products are represented in Canada by Nelson Education, Ltd.

For your lifelong learning solutions, visit **delmar.cengage.com**

Visit our corporate website at **www.cengage.com**

**Notice to the Reader**
Publisher does not warrant or guarantee any of the products described herein or perform any independent analysis in connection with any of the product information contained herein. Publisher does not assume, and expressly disclaims, any obligation to obtain and include information other than that provided to it by the manufacturer. The reader is expressly warned to consider and adopt all safety precautions that might be indicated by the activities described herein and to avoid all potential hazards. By following the instructions contained herein, the reader willingly assumes all risks in connection with such instructions. The publisher makes no representations or warranties of any kind, including but not limited to, the warranties of fitness for particular purpose or merchantability, nor are any such representations implied with respect to the material set forth herein, and the publisher takes no responsibility with respect to such material. The publisher shall not be liable for any special, consequential, or exemplary damages resulting, in whole or in part, from the readers' use of, or reliance upon, this material.

Printed in United States of America
12 13 14 15 16 17 15 14 13 12 11

# Contents

## CHAPTER 3    THE DISEASE PROCESS    31

**APPENDIX B    ANSWERS TO QUESTIONS
                FOR DISCUSSION                    186**

**APPENDIX C    GLOSSARY                          194**

**INDEX        205**

# Preface

*Basic Infection Control for Health Care Providers,* Second Edition, is designed to provide current, relevant information about infection control and infectious disease. Health care providers from any discipline and at any experience level will benefit from the practical advice contained in this book. Whether you are just starting out as a student in one of the many health-related professions or are an experienced health care provider, this book will give you the information you need to protect yourself from infectious disease and protect yourself from legal repercussions.

This book may also prove useful for others who have occupational exposure to blood and other potentially infectious material. Child care workers, police officers, firefighters, factory workers, and tattoo artists may all benefit from the material contained herein. Regardless of your occupation, this book will serve as a practical reference and a helpful tool.

Infection control is a dynamic field. Practically every month discoveries are made, court decisions are formed, and outbreaks are tracked. The future of infection control is exciting. Even as you read this, the Centers for Disease Control and Prevention, as well as state and local health officials, are monitoring emerging infectious diseases in an attempt to prevent outbreaks. Changes in this field come often, and have far-reaching consequences.

# DEVELOPMENT OF THIS BOOK

Several years ago I was given the opportunity to teach an infection control class for a multidisciplined group of health care providers. The challenge, I soon discovered, was finding an appropriate book for the class. Infection control books were available, but none that provided the breadth and depth of information that I wished to cover.

The solution, although not an optimal one, was to photocopy my many pages of notes for the students, adding to the material as I discovered topics that needed to be covered. This packet of notes developed into a small, self-published booklet that, after many classes of student review, served as a foundation for the first edition of *Basic Infection Control for Health Care Providers*. Much of the material in this book is a result of student critique of my self-published book.

In this, the second edition of *Basic Infection Control for Health Care Providers*, I have integrated suggestions and input from health care professionals in a variety of disciplines, making this edition more valuable to a greater number of health care professions, including:

- child care providers
- chiropractors
- dentists, dental assistants, and hygienists
- emergency medical services personnel
- fire service personnel
- industrial safety personnel
- laboratory personnel
- medical assistants
- nursing home workers
- nursing personnel
- occupational therapists

- physical therapy personnel
- physicians
- radiological technologists
- respiratory therapists and technicians
- shelter workers
- sports medicine personnel, coaches, and trainers
- teachers and school personnel
- workers in business and industry

# ORGANIZATION OF THE TEXT

*Basic Infection Control for Health Care Providers,* Second edition, includes eight chapters and three appendixes intended to provide the reader with a well-rounded package of materials in a convenient format.

The chapters are designed to give the reader background information on the history of infection control, legal issues, how the process of disease works, overview of the immune system, how to protect yourself in the workplace and from agents used as weapons, and what to do if you have been exposed to an infectious agent. The latter half of the book contains information an over 45 diseases including information on:

- causative agents
- body systems affected
- susceptibility
- routes of transmission
- signs and symptoms
- patient treatment
- protective measures
- immunizations
- incubation period

Readers will also find answers to discussion questions and a glossary.

# FEATURES OF THE BOOK

This book offers the following features:

*Learning Objectives*—Each chapter opens with a list of learning objectives that are the substance of the chapter content.

*Key Terms*—A listing of key terms alerts the reader to terms that may be new or unfamiliar. These terms are bolded in the text and defined in the glossary.

*Featured Case Studies*—Real-life case studies are used to illustrate key points followed by questions that promote critical thinking.

*Questions for Discussion*—Questions are based on learning objectives and answers may be found within the chapter or in Appendix B.

*Alerts*—Alerts are used to call attention to something about which the health care provider should be aware.

*Newsmaker*—This feature highlights notable occasions when infectious diseases have made the news. Critical Thinking Questions follow each Newsmaker feature.

*Web Resources*—Web resources provide the reader with additional resources for further study.

*Glossary*—The glossary provides definitions for more than 200 specialized terms.

*Infectious Disease Reference*—This reference, included as Appendix A, provides relevant, easy-to-read information on a number of infectious diseases.

These features, coupled with the content applicable to any of the health care disciplines, make this book one that is as comprehensive as it is easy to read.

# NEW TO THIS EDITION

*New Organization*—Diseases of Concern have moved from Chapter 5 to an Appendix, making the information easier to access.

*Featured Case Study*—Promotes critical thinking with scenarios based on real-life situations.

*Newsmaker*—Relates infection control information to actual occurrences that were publicized in the media.

*Under the Microscope*—Gives the reader a chance to delve deeper into the topics being discussed.

*Web Resources*—Have been completely updated!

# SUPPLEMENT PACKAGE

The *Instructor Manual* is designed to complement *Basic Infection Control for Health Care Providers* and create an integrated teaching package that will provide the instructor with resources needed to conduct an infection control course that exceeds OSHA standards.

The *Instructor Manual* includes:
- Chapter quizzes and a final exam
- Sample course agendas
- Course materials and resources
- Materials for exercises and role-plays

# ABOUT THE AUTHOR

Mike Kennamer is a graduate of the paramedic program at Gadsden State Community College in Gadsden, Alabama. He holds a B.S. in public safety administration from Athens State University in Athens, Alabama, and an M.P.A. from Jacksonville State University in Jacksonville, Alabama. He is currently pursuing an

Ed.D. in higher education administration at the University of Alabama.

Mr. Kennamer currently serves as director of workforce development at Northeast Alabama Community College, where he previously served as chair of the skills training division and director of the EMS department. Kennamer has authored several books and video series, and has contributed to a number of projects, including both print and web-based projects. His experience in teaching in and administering a variety of allied health programs gives him a strong foundation from which to write.

# ACKNOWLEDGMENTS

I wish to thank the following reviewers who provided valuable input on the content and structure of the second edition:

Susan Erue, RN, BSN, MS, PHDc
Iowa Wesleyan College
Mt. Pleasant, IA

Marie Moran, RN, SDC
Ft. Collins, CO

Spencer Parker, BSN, RN
Atlanta, GA

Pat Trapp, RN, MAE
Beaver Dam Community Hospital
Columbus, WI

Special thanks are due to Barbara Acello, RN, who served as technical reviewer for the second edition. Her help and input were invaluable.

I would also like to thank the reviewers of the first edition for their sage advice and input:

Ann Sims, RN, BSN
Albuquerque Technical-Vocational Institute
Albuquerque, NM

Rich Bronson, MEd, EMT-P
Oklahoma State Department of Health
Grove, OK

Nancy Bourgeois, RN, BSN
Office of Public Health
Baton Rouge, LA

I also wish to thank the many students and colleagues who have reviewed one or more chapters, made suggestions on content, or simply put up with my incessant questions about what should, and should not, be included in a book on infection control for health care providers.

The people on the Delmar Cengage Learning team have been wonderful. Special thanks are due to managing editor Marah Bellegarde for working with me to shape a vision for this second edition and to William Brottmiller and Matthew Kane for believing enough in this project to fund it. I appreciate all that Acquisitions Editor Matt Seeley has done to keep the project on track, and I thank production editor Anne Sherman, production director Carolyn Miller, copy editor Debbie Stone, and project manager Sonia Taneja for turning my manuscript pages and notes into the attractive book you are now holding. Although we did not work together on a daily basis, the efforts of marketing director, Jennifer McAvey and marketing manager, Michele McTighe are apparent and much appreciated.

As always, my family was instrumental to my ability to complete this book. Special thanks are due to my wife, Trisha, and sons, Devin, Cody, and Lane.

## FEEDBACK

The author is interested in hearing from anyone who would like to offer suggestions or constructive criticism for future editions of this book. Please feel free to contact the author through Delmar or directly by e-mail at mike@kennamer.net.

## CHAPTER 1

# Introduction to Infection Control

## LEARNING OBJECTIVES

After completing this chapter, the reader should be able to:

- discuss the history of infectious disease.
- discuss the history of infection control.
- recognize and discuss modern infection control threats.
- list three key figures in the development of modern infection control.
- recognize and discuss infection control as a rapidly changing field.

## KEY TERMS

- acquired immunodeficiency syndrome (AIDS)
- Centers for Disease Control and Prevention (CDC)
- chronically infected
- hepatitis B (HBV)
- hepatitis C (HCV)
- hygiene
- occupational exposure
- tuberculosis (TB)
- virulence

## FEATURED CASE STUDY

Date:        November 13, 1738
Patient:     Miss Musgrave
Physician:   Dr. William Brownrigg

Miss Musgrave, a spotty, delicate girl, suffers from a serious fever. Her face is puffy and swollen, the puffiness having first appeared on her forehead and spread downward to her nose, upper lips, and cheeks. She reports severe pain in her face and her urine is pale.

Complicating the fact that Miss Musgrave has a delicate constitution, the weather has been excessively wet and rainy and moist and cold with Westerly winds. This has caused the patient's humours [fluids] to become corrupted and imbalanced.

She was bled seven times within six days. A large quantity was obtained each time, causing the patient to feel faint. Local plasters of nitrous powders and tartar were applied to the back of the neck and lower legs and she was given a suitable cooling diet.

1. Based on the notes provided in Dr. Brownrigg's casebook, we can begin to form a clinical opinion of his patient's condition. What do you expect that Miss Musgrave's diagnosis would be today?
2. Eighteenth-century physicians were convinced that an imbalance of fluids (blood, phlegm, bile, urine, and sweat) caused illness and that the only way to cure the patient was to rid the body of noxious fluids. How would Miss Musgrave's treatment differ today from that in 1738?

# INTRODUCTION

Infection control is a rapidly changing field. This book is an overview of how the health care provider who is at risk of **occupational exposure** to blood and/or body fluid may be protected from contracting a communicable disease. Persons reading this book should realize that because changes occur rapidly, the instructor of this course is an important resource for the most up-to-date information.

# HISTORY OF INFECTIOUS DISEASE

Although the cause of infections was not well understood until later, people have known of and studied infections for many years. Ancient texts written as early as 1450 BC describe signs of infections.

> When someone has a swelling or a blister or a shiny spot on the skin that might signal a serious skin disease on the body, bring him to Aaron the priest or to one of his priest sons. The priest will examine the sore on the skin. If the hair in the sore has turned white and the sore appears more than skin deep, it is a serious skin disease and infectious.
>
> Leviticus 13:2-3a
> The Message

Approximately one thousand years later, around 450 BC, early scholars recorded the life of King Asa of Judah including his suffering and dying from a foot infection.

> A full account of Asa is written in The Chronicles of the Kings of Judah. In the thirty-ninth year of his reign Asa came down with a severe case of foot infection. He didn't ask GOD for help, but went instead to the doctors. Then Asa died; he died in the forty-first year of his reign.
>
> 2 Chronicles 16:11-13
> The Message

Greek physician Hippocrates indicated that the ancient Greeks studied and sought the origins of infectious diseases as early as 400 BC. Hippocrates wrote of the dangers posed by stagnant pools of water and expressed the importance of good **hygiene** in promoting good health.

> From these things he must proceed to investigate everything else. For if one knows all these things well, or at least the greater part of them, he cannot miss knowing, when he comes into a strange city, either the diseases peculiar to the place, or the particular nature of common diseases, so that he will not be in doubt as to the treatment of the diseases, or commit mistakes, as is likely to be the case provided one had not previously considered these matters.
>
> Hippocrates, in
> Airs, Waters, and Places

The ancient Romans built elaborate systems of aqueducts, which helped to promote health and sanitation. By 97 AD the Romans had constructed nine aqueducts, mainly to provide water for bathing and drinking. By 226 AD Roman aqueducts were discharging nearly 300 million gallons of water each day.

As a result of the survival of reports of the French Inquisition, evidence of hygienic practices among 13th-century medieval peasants exists. In Montaillou, a village in the mountains of southern France, reports indicate that hardly anyone, rich or poor, ever had a bath. Only the hands and mouth—those parts of the body involved in preparing, blessing, or consuming food—were kept relatively clean. It was not until the mid-17th century that theories regarding germs and disease became accurate.

## HISTORY OF MODERN INFECTION CONTROL

Modern infection control ideas originated in Vienna, Austria, in the mid-1800s when a physician, Ignaz Semmelweis, discovered that hand washing seemed to decrease the incidence of death due to infection following childbirth. By observing simple hand washing procedures, the death rate related to infection decreased from

18% to 1% in Semmelweis's hospital. Although Semmelweis was excited with his discovery, the concept of washing hands before and after medical procedures was not routinely practiced until much later.

Unfortunately, Semmelweis's colleagues were not as enthusiastic about his discovery. His hospital censured him and reduced his privileges. When he reported his findings to the Medical Society of Vienna, he met enough resistance to lead him to his native Budapest. There he was committed to an insane asylum, where he died of an infection similar to those he had tried to prevent in Austria.

During about the same period, French scientist Louis Pasteur created his germ theory. A background in physics and chemistry led Pasteur to approach the study of microbial life in a different way. Pasteur believed that microbes can bring about significant transformations in organic matter—transformations that are very selective and specific in their activities. Pasteur also discovered anaerobic life when practical application of his germ theory proved that, in the absence of air, sugar was converted to butyric acid. Not only did his different approach open new doors in the field of microbiology, it also led to the development of the process of pasteurization—a technique of controlled heating for the preservation of various food products.

Scottish surgeon Joseph Lister expanded Pasteur's germ theory by using cotton wool and bandages treated with carbolic acid to dress surgical wounds. It was Lister who discovered that infection could be prevented by covering wounds and using antiseptic agents. Like Semmelweis, the efficacy of Lister's work was demonstrated by a postsurgery mortality rate that decreased from 50% to 15%. And like Semmelweis, he initially experienced great resistance from the medical community. Lister, however, persevered and became famous during his lifetime. He performed surgery on Queen Victoria and opened the way for techniques of modern surgery.

Just as Semmelweis had trouble convincing his colleagues to wash their hands, health care providers as recently as several years ago were not convinced of the necessity of observing standard precautions against communicable disease. What do you think it took to convince health care providers to observe precautions against communicable disease? See if you agree with the analysis in the following section.

## INFECTION CONTROL BECOMES AN ISSUE

In the 1980s, a disease called **acquired immunodeficiency syndrome (AIDS)** was introduced to the American public. Although early reports sparked little interest, people began to take note when celebrities and sports figures became infected with the disease. As word of the disease spread throughout the country, persons with occupational exposure to blood started to routinely wear gloves and other protective equipment. At the time, little was known about AIDS and its causative agent, human immunodeficiency virus (HIV).

Organizations set standards and the U.S. government began work on legislation that would protect America's health care workers.

Hepatitis B virus (HBV) emerged as a considerable health risk during the late 1980s and early 1990s. Although HIV is a deadly virus, it does not survive well outside the human body. Conversely, HBV can survive for hours or even days outside the human body, posing a greater risk to health care professionals. Although a vaccine for HBV was developed as early as 1971, it was

# NEWSMAKER
## Johnson Infected Retires

LOS ANGELES, CA                                   NOVEMBER 7, 1991

On November 7, 1991, Earvin "Magic" Johnson announced his retirement from the Los Angeles Lakers. The 6-ft. 9-in. tall, 32-year-old NBA star was at the pinnacle of his career. He was loved by the fans and respected by his fellow players. Johnson told the reporters gathered at the Great Western Forum in Los Angeles that he had been infected with the HIV virus and would "have to retire from the Lakers today."

The announcement was shocking. "When you look at a big, healthy guy like Magic Johnson," said Keven McHale of the Boston Celtics, "you think this illness wouldn't attack someone like him." But it did.

"We think sometimes it can only happen to gay people, it can't happen to me," said Johnson, who, it is believed, contracted HIV through heterosexual contact. "And here I am saying it can happen to anybody, even me, Magic Johnson."

Johnson's revelation brought the issue of AIDS and infectious diseases in general to the forefront of popular culture. Once considered a disease that affected only those in developing countries, or homosexuals, or intravenous drug users, HIV now had a face in Magic Johnson. The part that frightened the public was that they could relate to Johnson. No longer was HIV an "awful disease" affecting this group or that group. HIV had hit home.

1. Why do you think media coverage of HIV had been limited until Magic Johnson's announcement?

2. How did Magic Johnson's forthrighness about his condition help prompt the public to learn more about HIV and AIDS?

3. Do you think that the media coverage given to HIV and AIDS helped increase the public's awareness of infectious disease in general?

4. What other infectious diseases have been brought to public attention through the media in recent years?

## UNDER THE MICROSCOPE

❂ Research Magic Johnson's life since his Novermber 7, 1991, announcement. What is his current status? What has he done to support awareness of HIV and AIDS?

❂ List and discuss others who have increased public awareness of communicable diseases.

❂ As a health care provider you will be seen as an authority in your own community. Discuss how you can help increase public awareness of infection control in your own neighborhood.

❂   ❂   ❂

not widely used. In 1981 the U.S. Food and Drug Administration (FDA) approved the first commercial HBV vaccine. This vaccine was derived from protective antibodies contained in the blood of patients who had recovered from a hepatitis B infection. The widespread use of this vaccine and its second-generation genetically engineered synthetic successor, approved in 1986, helped to quell the increase in numbers of those infected with HBV.

### ALERT

Diseases other than hepatitis and human immunodeficiency virus (HIV) pose a risk for health care providers. Always protect yourself from all infectious and communicable disease.

## CURRENT PERSPECTIVE

Today communicable disease is taken seriously. Employees take the initiative to better protect themselves and employers meet stringent standards imposed by the federal government to ensure a safe workplace.

AIDS remains a formidable disease, for which there is no vaccine and no cure. However, other diseases, such as **tuberculosis (TB)**, **hepatitis B (HBV)**, and **hepatitis C (HCV)** continue to affect health care providers and remain considerable health risks. Although the number of new HBV infections has declined from 260,000 per year in the 1980s to about 73,000 per year in 2003, an estimated 1.25 million Americans remain chronically infected with HBV.

It is estimated that 3.9 million Americans have been infected with HCV, 2.7 million of whom are **chronically infected**, which means that they will always be infected. Because of the **virulence**, or the degree of its ability to cause a disease, of hepatitis and its ability to survive outside the confines of the human body, health care providers are at risk of occupational exposure.

# STATISTICS

The United Nations estimates that nearly 38 million people worldwide are infected with HIV, the virus that causes AIDS. An estimated 950,000 of these are U.S. residents and, according to the **Centers for Disease Control and Prevention (CDC)**, the component of the U.S. Department of Health and Human Services instrumental in setting infection control standards, 180,000 to 280,000 are unaware that they are infected.

Hepatitis B emerged as a significant health risk in the 1980s. Although public education and an effective vaccine have contributed to decreasing numbers of persons infected with hepatitis B virus (HBV), the CDC estimates that 78,000 U.S. residents become infected each year. Hepatitis B is very environmentally resistant and can survive for long periods of time, even outside the body.

Currently, hepatitis C is the most common chronic bloodborne infection in the United States. An estimated 3.9 million Americans have been infected with HCV. Worldwide, it is estimated that 350 million have been infected. According to the CDC, most of these persons may not be aware of their infection because they are not clinically ill.

Work on an HCV vaccine is ongoing; however, development has been difficult. Traditional means of vaccine development have been unsuccessful, since unlike hepatitis A or B, antibodies to hepatitis C even at high levels do not lead to recovery and fail to prevent current or subsequent infection. Research continues in this important quest.

Other diseases may pose a risk to the health care provider. **Tuberculosis (TB)**, which was once the leading cause of death in the United States, was thought to be a disease of the past until 1984, when it began to make a comeback. Many attribute the comeback of tuberculosis to public apathy and failure to vaccinate.

## INFECTED HEALTH CARE WORKERS

Although health care providers are at risk of occupational exposure to blood and body fluids, their risk of actually contracting an infection is fairly low. For instance, the annual number of occupational HBV infections was fewer than 400 in 2001. This is a significant decrease from the more than 10,000 new cases involving occupational exposure in health care in 1983. Today, health care personnel who have received HBV vaccine and in whom immunity has developed are at virtually no risk for infection. Although there is a risk for infection from exposures of mucous membranes or nonintact skin, there is no known risk from exposure of intact skin. The risk from a single needlestick or cut exposure to HBV-infected blood ranges from 6 to 30%, depending on the antigen status of the source individual.

No exact estimates on the number of occupational exposures to HCV in the health care industry are available; however, studies have shown that 1% of hospital health care personnel have evidence of HCV infection, compared with 3% of the overall U.S. population. Studies also reveal that 2% of health care workers will become infected with HCV after an exposure to HCV-infected blood or a needlestick involving HCV-infected blood.

Occupational exposure to HIV is rare. However, HIV continues to be an international concern, especially in developing countries. From 1985 to 2001, the CDC reported 57 documented cases and 138 possible cases of occupationally acquired HIV infection among health care personnel in the United States. The average risk of HIV infection after a needlestick or cut exposure to HIV-infected blood is 0.3% (1 in 300). Stated another way, 99.7% of needlestick/cut exposures to HIV-infected blood do not lead to infection. The risk after exposure of the eye, mouth, or nose to HIV-infected blood is estimated to be 1 in 1000 (0.1%). The risk after short-term exposure to intact skin is nil, whereas the risk after exposure to nonintact skin is less than 0.1%.

## INTERESTING FACTS

- There is no known risk of HBV, HCV, or HIV from exposure of intact skin.
- Only 1% of hospital health care personnel have evidence of HCV infection, versus 3% of the general U.S. population.

## INTERESTING FACTS (continued)

- 98% of those exposed to HCV-infected blood through a needlestick or cut exposure will not become infected.
- 99.7% of those exposed to HIV-infected blood through a needlestick or cut exposure will not become infected.
- 99.9% of those exposed to HIV-infected blood through exposure of nonintact skin or mucous membranes of the mouth, eye, or nose will not become infected.

## CONCLUSION

All health care providers have an obligation to learn about infectious disease in an effort to protect themselves and their patients. The remainder of this book will serve as a basis for that knowledge.

## QUESTIONS FOR DISCUSSION

1. What diseases have increased public awareness of infection control over the past few years?
2. What simple infection control procedure helped Dr. Ignaz Semmelweis save a number of lives in the 1800s?
3. List three pioneers in the field of infection control.
4. List at least three diseases that should concern health care workers today.
5. Explain how we know that ancient civilizations knew of and were concerned about infectious diseases.

## WORTH THINKING ABOUT

- Try to recall the first time you heard about AIDS. Have you experienced prejudices against those with AIDS or other communicable diseases? Why?

- Have you ever cared for a person with AIDS? Did you take more precautions with this patient than you normally do? Why?

## WEB RESOURCES

**Centers for Disease Control and Prevention**—This site provides a wealth of information on infectious disease, infection control, and statistics. Click on MMWR (Morbidity and Mortality Weekly Report) for detailed trends and statistics. http://www.cdc.gov.

**Association for Professionals in Infection Control and Epidemiology (APIC)**—This is the official site of the premier organization for infection-control professionals. http://www.apic.org.

## BIBLIOGRAPHY

Centers for Disease Control and Prevention. (2003). *Exposure to blood: What healthcare personnel need to know.* Atlanta: Author.

Centers for Disease Control and Prevention. (2006). *Hepatitis B fact sheet.* Atlanta: Author.

Centers for Disease Control and Prevention. (2003). *Hepatitis C fact sheet.* Atlanta: Author.

Dubos, R. J., & Hirsch, J. G. (1965). *Bacterial and mycotic infections of man.* Philadelphia: Lippincott.

Hippocrates. (400 BC). *On airs, waters, and places.* Accessed April 15, 2006, from http://www.4literature.net.

Hoofnagle, J. H. (2004). *Testimony before the Committee on Government Reform of the United States House of Representatives.* Washington, DC: U.S. Department of Health and Human Services.

Joint United Nations Programme on HIV/AIDS. (2004). *2004 Report on the global AIDS epidemic.* Geneva, Switzerland: Author.

Peterson, E. (2002) *The message: The Bible in contemporary language.* Colorado Springs: NavPress Publishing.

Shimeld, L. A., & Rodgers, A. T. (1999). *Essentials of diagnostic microbiology.* Clifton Park, NY: Thomson Delmar Learning.

Waller, J. (2002). *The discovery of the germ.* Cambridge, U.K.: Icon Books.

## CHAPTER 2

# Legal Issues

## LEARNING OBJECTIVES

After completing this chapter, the reader should be able to:

- list at least four things required by the OSHA bloodborne pathogen standard.
- explain the importance of meeting accepted standards.
- discuss the intent of the Ryan White CARE Act.
- describe the role of the designated officer.
- list at least three organizations that are considered leaders in infection control issues.
- describe reasons for learning more about infection control.
- list the components of a successful negligence lawsuit.

## KEY TERMS

- Americans with Disabilities Act (ADA)
- American Institute of Architects (AIA)
- Association for Professionals in Infection Control and Epidemiology (APIC)
- breach of duty
- category I employee
- Centers for Disease Control and Prevention (CDC)
- civil liability
- damages
- designated officer

- duty to act
- essential functions
- exposure control plan
- Joint Commission on Accreditation of Healthcare Organizations (JCAHO)
- negligence
- notification by request
- Occupational Safety and Health Administration (OSHA)
- Other Than Serious Violation
- proximate cause
- qualified individual with a disability
- reasonable accommodations
- Repeat Violation
- routine notification
- Ryan White CARE Act of 1990
- Serious Violation
- standard of care
- undue hardship
- Willful Violation

## ☀ FEATURED CASE STUDY ☀

Date:        September 16, 1994
Patient:     Ms. Sydney Abbott
Dentist:     Dr. Randon Bragdon

Sydney Abbott visited the office of Dr. Randon Bragdon, a Bangor, Maine, dentist. While completing a routine medical history form, Abbott indicated that she was infected with HIV, though she was asymptomatic.

Because she was infected with HIV, Dr. Bragdon refused to fill Ms. Abbott's cavity in his office but offered to perform the procedure in a local hospital, a facility better equipped to treat HIV patients, at Abbott's expense.

Believing that she had been discriminated against, Abbott sued her dentist for discrimination under the Americans with Disabilities Act (ADA). Bragdon, she contended, had discriminated against her because of a disability. The district court and the U.S. Court of Appeals for the First Circuit granted summary judgment to the plaintiff on the grounds that her condition constituted a disability under ADA and that treating her in the defendant's office would not have posed a direct threat to the safety and health of others. Nearly 4 years later, on June 25, 1998, the U.S. Supreme Court agreed that HIV is a qualifying disability under ADA and remanded the case back to the First Circuit asking the lower court to determine if the plaintiff's HIV infection posed a direct threat to the defendant.

1. The Supreme Court determined that the presence of HIV is a qualifying disability under the ADA since it substantially limits one or more major life activities, including the ability to reproduce. List other major life activities that may be limited when a person has an infectious disease.
2. The case was sent back to the lower court to determine if Abbott's asymptomatic HIV infection posed a threat to Dr. Bragdon. According to Bragdon, as of September 1994, the Centers for Disease Control and Prevention (CDC) had identified seven dental workers with suspected occupational transmission of HIV. Do you believe that the plaintiff's HIV infection posed a threat to the defendant?

## UNDER THE MICROSCOPE

❖ Search the Internet or your local law library to learn if there have been other ADA cases related to infectious disease. Discuss your findings.

❖ In what way do you suppose the hospital was better able, according to Dr. Bragdon, to care for a patient with HIV? What precautions should be taken in any setting?

# INTRODUCTION

It is important to learn about infection control for any number of reasons. This chapter describes three. First, administrative law requires that employees at risk of occupational exposure to blood and body fluids receive training on infection control issues. Second, those who fail to meet established standards may be subject to civil action. And third, most people want to learn about infection control to protect their personal health and that of others. By applying infection control practices, health care providers not only learn to protect themselves, they also learn to protect those with whom they come into contact.

# OCCUPATIONAL SAFETY AND HEALTH ADMINISTRATION

In 1991, the **Occupational Safety and Health Administration (OSHA),** under authority of Congress, set the rule for occupational exposure to bloodborne pathogens in title 29, part 1910 of the Code of Federal Regulations. This rule was a landmark in the development of infection-control programs in the United States and set the wheels in motion for the development of infection control education as it is known today.

Each agency's exposure-control plan should be tailored for the agency. Common components of the plan should include:

✳ Purpose

✳ Scope (To whom does the plan apply?)

✳ Exposure determination

✳ Postexposure protocols

✳ Standard operating procedures

✳ Roles and responsibilities

✳ Personal protective equipment

✳ Training standards

✳ Health maintenance

✳ Engineering controls

✳ Compliance and quality monitoring

**FIGURE 2-1** Exposure control plan contents. (*Source:* Occupational Safety and Health Administration.)

This rule identified health care providers and emergency response personnel as **category I employees,** who are at the greatest risk of occupational exposure to communicable disease. It also mandated each employer with category I employees to develop an **exposure control plan** and to offer hepatitis B vaccinations at no charge to the employee. Standards on personal protective equipment (PPE), recordkeeping, training, and work practices were also developed and carry the weight of law. Required exposure control plan contents are listed in Figure 2-1.

Federal law requires that states comply with OSHA regulations or develop a plan that meets or exceeds OSHA standards. To see if your state has an approved OSHA plan, see Figure 2-2.

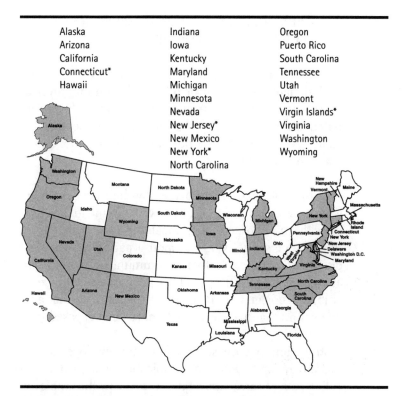

| Alaska | Indiana | Oregon |
| Arizona | Iowa | Puerto Rico |
| California | Kentucky | South Carolina |
| Connecticut* | Maryland | Tennessee |
| Hawaii | Michigan | Utah |
| | Minnesota | Vermont |
| | Nevada | Virgin Islands* |
| | New Jersey* | Virginia |
| | New Mexico | Washington |
| | New York* | Wyoming |
| | North Carolina | |

**FIGURE 2-2** States and territories with OSHA-approved plans. (*Source:* Occupational Safety and Health Administration.)
*Plans cover public sector employment only.

 **ALERT**

It is your responsibility to be aware of the content of your agency's exposure control plan.

## RYAN WHITE CARE ACT

Another law that applies to some health care workers is the **Ryan White Comprehensive AIDS Resources Emergency (CARE) Act of 1990**. This law, reauthorized in 1996 and 2000, gives emergency response personnel the right to learn if they were exposed to an infectious disease while caring for a patient.

The law requires the public health officer of each state to designate one official or officer of each employer of emergency response personnel in the state. This **designated officer** serves as a liaison between the medical facility and the affected personnel. Notification takes place in one of two ways.

**Routine notification** is provided by the medical facility to employees exposed to a patient who is found to be infected with an airborne communicable disease. Emergency response personnel who transport a patient who is later discovered to have an airborne communicable disease are automatically considered to have been exposed. Since an ambulance is an enclosed space, it is assumed that anyone within that space is likely to have been exposed.

**Notification by request** is made by any employee who is potentially exposed to a communicable disease while providing patient care. This request is made by the employee and coordinated through the designated officer.

## AMERICANS WITH DISABILITIES ACT

The **Americans with Disabilities Act (ADA)** is intended to prohibit discrimination against persons with disabilities. The act specifically notes "contagious disease" as a qualifying disability, which ensures that employees who contract a communicable disease will not be discriminated against.

### Employment

To be covered under the ADA an employer must engage in an industry affecting commerce and have 15 or more employees each working day in each of 20 or more calendar weeks in the current or preceding year. Employers exempt from the ADA include Indian tribes and corporations wholly owned by the U.S. government.

The ADA prohibits employers from discriminating against **qualified individuals with a disability** in any of the following areas:

- Hiring, advancement, and discharge of employees
- Job training
- Employee compensation

A qualified individual with a disability is one who meets the requisite skill, education, experience, and other job-related requirements of the position the individual holds or desires and who, with or without **reasonable accommodations,** can perform the **essential functions** of the job.

The essential functions of a job are those fundamental duties that must be performed unaided or with the assistance of a reasonable accommodation. These functions are those considered fundamental to the job. A reasonable accommodation is a modification to the work environment that enables a person with a disability to perform the essential functions of a job. If an accommodation causes an **undue hardship**—that is, an action requiring significant expense or difficulty to an employer— the employer may legally refuse to provide the accommodation under the terms of the ADA.

## Public Accommodations and Commercial Facilities

The ADA also provides equal access to public accommodations and commercial facilities. This means that, according to the law, individuals "shall not be discriminated against on the basis of disability in the full and equal enjoyment of the goods, services, facilities, privileges, advantages, or accommodations of any place of public accommodation." The professional office of a health care provider is considered a place of public accommodation. As such, health care providers are prohibited from discriminating against individuals on the basis of their disabilities, as illustrated in this chapter's case study.

## NEEDLESTICK PREVENTION AND SAFETY ACT

The Centers for Disease Control and Prevention (CDC) estimate that up to 800,000 percutaneous injuries from contaminated sharps occur each year among U.S. health care workers. To help address this problem, Congress passed the Needlestick Prevention and Safety Act of 2000. This act, which enjoyed strong bipartisan support, was signed into law on November 6, 2000. Its purpose is to protect health care providers from accidental needlesticks by requiring employers to solicit input from non-managerial employees, responsible for direct patient care, in the identification, evaluation, and selection of effective engineering and work practice controls. Specific provisions of this act include an emphasis on selection, training, and use of safer medical devices and the development of a sharps injury log for better surveillance of percutaneous injuries from contaminated sharps.

This log is required in addition to the OSHA 300 log and must contain the following items:

- the type and brand of device involved in the incident
- the work area or department where the incident occurred
- an explanation of how the incident occurred

Companies who have employed no more than 10 employees at any time during the preceding calendar year are not required to maintain this log. The information on this log must be kept for 5 years and maintained in such a way as to protect the confidentiality of the injured employee.

# NEWSMAKER
## Ryan White Dies at 18

CICERO, IN                                      APRIL 8, 1990

Ryan White, the young man who emerged as a powerful voice for AIDS prevention and treatment in the late 1980s died today. He was 18 years old.

It was the day after Christmas in 1984 when then 13-year-old Ryan White was told by his mother that he had AIDS. A hemophiliac, White had become infected through a transfusion of HIV-tainted blood and later became an important force in educating the public about AIDS.

A young boy with a misunderstood disease, Ryan White was often the victim of fear and ignorance. Children in school called him names and ostracized him. Adults refused to shake hands with his family at church, and someone even fired a bullet into his house. Frightened parents asked that Ryan be kept out of school, and Ryan sued to secure his right to a public education. Although he won the suit, he still felt uncomfortable in his hometown of Kokomo, Indiana, so he moved to Cicero, Indiana, where he was welcomed at Hamilton Heights High School.

It was during his legal battle that Ryan White decided to dedicate the remainder of his life to educating the public about AIDS. Until his death today, Ryan White captivated Americans with his knowledge of and courage in dealing with his disease.

Ryan White's contribution to public education about AIDS was essential in building a foundation of understanding and helping to dispel many myths about the disease. This contribution prompted Congress to name the most comprehensive AIDS legislation to date after Ryan White, a young man who demanded the attention and respect of all who heard him speak.

1. What do you believe motivated people to discriminate against Ryan White?

2. Why is Ryan White such an important figure to: The HIV/AIDS community? The health care community? The disabled?

## UNDER THE MICROSCOPE

- Search the Internet for Hamilton Heights High School. Visit the Media Center to find a link to the Ryan White archives. Consider how Ryan White's high school experience was similar to, and different from, yours.
- Conduct research to learn the effect Ryan White had on the world. What can you do to be a positive influence in your family, school, state, country, world?

# AGENCIES AND REGULATIONS

Several agencies have established standards for infection control. The **Centers for Disease Control and Prevention (CDC)** has been instrumental in publishing standards for infection control and in establishing guidelines for standard precautions. The CDC tracks selected diseases and monitors for trends in the appearance of diseases in a particular area. Through research, education, and extensive publishing in the area of infectious disease, the CDC has emerged as an incredible resource for those who wish to learn more about infection control.

The **Joint Commission on Accreditation of Healthcare Organizations (JCAHO)** has been a leader in developing standards for health and safety in health care delivery. JCAHO infection control standards require that health care organizations develop and implement plans to control infection, monitor the presence of and spread of infection, and take the necessary steps to control infection. JCAHO released revised infection control standards in 2003, which became effective in January 2005.

Other organizations have established standards on infection control. The **American Institute of Architects (AIA)** has established guidelines for engineering infection control safety into the construction of health care facilities. The **Association for Professionals in Infection Control and Epidemiology (APIC)** has published standards and practice guidelines on a variety of infection control topics and is an established leader in many facets of infection control. Other organizations, including state and local health departments, provide important and timely information related to infection control and emerging infectious diseases.

# CIVIL LIABILITY

Standards set forth by organizations may not carry the weight of law, but one should take these standards as seriously as if they were federal law.

Employers and/or employees may be found guilty of **civil liability** if damages occur as a result of not meeting recognized standards. Although no law is broken, they may be found negligent if they do not meet standards that would be met by another reasonable person in a similar position.

There are four components needed to prove that a health care provider was negligent. These four components of **negligence** are explained as follows:

- **Duty to act**—Before a person may be considered negligent, he/she must have a legal duty to provide care. This duty to act obligates the caregiver to treat the patient with the same **standard of care** that would be offered by another reasonable caregiver of the same level of education or licensure.
- **Breach of duty**—A breach of duty means that the caregiver did not meet his/her obligation in some way. This may be inappropriate care, abandonment, or care that is either above or below the caregiver's expected level of care.

- **Damages**—When a patient has experienced monetary loss, injury, or death, she or her family is said to have experienced damages. Damages may be tangible, like loss of income, or intangible, like loss of vision.
- **Proximate cause**—The final component that must be proven to show negligence is proximate cause. That is, that the damages resulted from the caregiver's breach of duty. Even if there are damages and a breach of duty, negligence is not proven until it can be shown that the damages were caused by the breach of duty.

Although we usually think of breach of duty as inappropriate action or treatment, it is possible that failure to meet accepted standards may constitute negligence when damages occur as a result of that failure.

## PERSONAL AND COMMUNITY HEALTH

Health care providers should, even if not required by law, seek to stay current with infection control training as a method of promoting personal health and the health of their families. Knowledge of infection control procedures and protection measures may contribute to a longer and more productive career and life.

Employees also have a responsibility to the community to learn how to minimize the possibility for cross contamination from patient-to-patient and from employee-to-patient. Health care providers who have young children should take an active role in educating neighborhood children of the importance of hand washing and the dangers of behavior that may lead to disease spread.

## CONCLUSION

There are a number of good reasons for learning more about infection control. Some people see legal repercussions as a good reason, while others are motivated by the desire to protect themselves and their families. Whatever your reason for learning, it is important that you stay up-to-date on infection control issues.

OSHA requires refresher training each year to keep health care providers up-to-date. Don't depend on taking one course or reading one book to keep you updated for life. Infection control is a dynamic field and should be revisited often, as scientific discoveries are made and legal cases are upheld or overturned. This is an area in which lifelong learning could prove to be a lifesaving experience.

## INTERESTING FACTS

OSHA may levy fines based on the following schedule:

- **Other Than Serious Violation** — A violation that has a direct relationship to safety and health, but is not likely to cause death or serious physical injury is categorized as "other than serious." A proposed penalty of up to $7000 may be levied.

- **Serious Violation** — A violation for which there is substantial probability that death or physical harm could result, and that the employer knew, or should have known, that the hazard existed. The penalty is $7000 per occurrence.

- **Willful Violation** — A willful violation is one that an employer knowingly commits or commits with indifference to the law. The penalty for each violation is $5000 to $70,000.

- **Repeat Violation** — A violation of any standard, rule, or order for which, upon reinspection, the same or a similar violation is found may result in a penalty of up to $70,000 for a repeat violation.

## INTERESTING FACTS (continued)

Inspections in the health care industry have resulted in the following penalties:

○ An ambulance service in Massachusetts was fined more than $60,000 because of failure to provide all required safeguards, including hepatitis B vaccine, to its employees.

○ A New York nursing home was fined $62,200 for repeat and serious violations involving the safety and health of their employees, including bloodborne pathogens standards.

○ A commercial laundry in New York received initial penalties of more than $140,000 for failing to protect employees against exposure to bloodborne pathogens.

○ A Connecticut hospital faced penalties of $91,500 for a variety of hazards, including those associated with bloodborne pathogens and respiratory protection.

○ A Georgia commercial laundry that provides laundry services to health care facilities was fined $50,000 for potentially exposing employees to bloodborne pathogens and not providing accessible sharps containers.

*Source:* Occupational Safety and Health Administration.


## QUESTIONS FOR DISCUSSION

1. List three things required by OSHA regarding infection control.
2. What is the intent of the Ryan White CARE Act?
3. Differentiate between states covered under state plans and states covered under federal OSHA jurisdiction.
4. List four components of a successful negligence lawsuit.

5. Describe the intent of the Americans with Disabilities Act (ADA).

6. Explain why it is important to meet standards recognized by leading agencies in the infection control field.

## WORTH THINKING ABOUT

- Consider the responsibility you feel in taking this course.
- How can your actions at work affect the health and safety of your family?
- Consider how you would feel if you were denied service or employment because of a disability.

## WEB RESOURCES

**Hamilton Heights High School Media Center**—This is the site for the Ryan White Digital Archive. http://www.library.riverturn.org.

**Americans with Disabilities Act site**—This is the official Department of Justice site containing information about the ADA. http://www.ada.gov.

**Occupational Safety and Health Administration**—OSHA's official site contains a plethora of information related to occupational safety and health. Visit their site at http://www.osha.gov.

## BIBLIOGRAPHY

*Abbott v. Bragdon*, 107 F3d 934 (1998).

American Society for Healthcare Engineering. (2005). *AIA guidelines for infection control*. Chicago: Author.

Centers for Disease Control and Prevention. (2004). *Worker health chartbook*. Atlanta: Author.

Channaiah, D. *The Ryan White story: A shift from confusion, fear, and ignorance to acceptance and new-found knowledge of AIDS*. http://www.engl.virginia.edu.

Joint Commission on Accreditation of Healthcare Organizations. (2004). *Setting the standard.* Oakbrook Terrace, IL: Author.

National Fire Academy. (1992). *Infection control for emergency response personnel: The supervisor's role.* Emmitsburg, MD: Author.

Nielson, R. P. (2000). *OSHA regulations and guidelines: A guide for health care providers.* Clifton Park, NY: Thomson Delmar Learning.

Occupational Safety and Health Administration. (2005). *State occupational safety and health plans.* http://www.osha.gov.

*Ryan White CARE Act of 1990.* U.S. Public Law 101-381.

*Ryan White CARE Act Amendments of 1996.* US Public Law 104-146.

*Ryan White CARE Act Amendments of 2000.* US Public Law 106-345.

U.S. Department of Justice. (2005). *ADA Regulations and Technical Assistance Materials.* http://www.usdoj.gov.

U.S. Department of Labor, Occupational Safety and Health Administration. (1991, Dec. 6). *Occupational exposure to bloodborne pathogens.* CFR 1910.1030, Final Rule: as amended at 57 FR 12717, April 13, 1992; 57 FR 29206, July 1, 1992; 61 FR 5507, Feb. 13, 1996; 66 FR 5325 Jan. 18, 2001.

## CHAPTER 3

# The Disease Process

## LEARNING OBJECTIVES

After completing this chapter, the reader should be able to:

- differentiate between infectious and communicable disease.
- describe at least two ways disease is spread.
- list at least four causes of infectious disease.
- list the stages of an infectious disease.
- explain the principles of seroconversion.

## KEY TERMS

- airborne transmission
- bacteria
- bloodborne transmission
- casual contact
- communicable disease
- communicable period
- disease period
- fungus
- helminths
- household contact
- incubation period
- infectious disease
- latent period

- other potentially infectious material (OPIM)
- parasitic
- protozoans
- rickettsia
- saprophytic
- seroconversion
- sexual transmission
- sexually transmitted disease (STD)
- vector-borne transmission
- virus
- window phase

## FEATURED CASE STUDY

Date:        June 12, 1999
Patient:     Ms. Phoebe Mayow
Physician:   Dr. Ezekiel Katz

Ms. Mayow, a 15-year-old female, presents to the emergency department accompanied by her mother. She reports becoming ill after returning from cheerleading camp. Currently she reports nausea, vomiting, abdominal cramping, and bloody diarrhea. Her skin is pale and cool.

Her mother, who picked her up at camp, tells you that the conditions at the camp were less than sanitary. "There was a barrel in her dormitory lobby filled with ice," reported Mrs. Mayow. "There were leaves and pieces of grass floating in the barrel," she continued. Phoebe told her mother that the girls filled their water bottles from that barrel and that some of the campers dipped their arms and hands in the barrel. One, according to Phoebe, even dipped her head in the barrel after an especially long practice session.

1. What is the likely source of the patient's illness?
2. How could this exposure have been prevented?
3. Would you expect to see additional patients with similar symptoms?
4. How could education have prevented this exposure?
5. Using the chain of infection shown in Figure 3-3, discuss ways the chain of infection could have been broken in this circumstance.

# INTRODUCTION

The material presented in this chapter forms a brief overview of the disease process. By understanding how the disease process works, health care providers can better protect themselves from infectious disease.

# DIFFERENTIATION OF INFECTIOUS AND COMMUNICABLE DISEASES

In the study of the disease process, it is important to differentiate between infectious disease and communicable disease (Figure 3-1). An **infectious disease** is one that results

| Infectious diseases that are communicable | Infectious diseases that are not communicable |
| --- | --- |
| ✳ Hepatitis B | ✳ Anthrax |
| ✳ Influenza | ✳ Botulism |
| ✳ Chlamydia | ✳ Salmonellosis |
| ✳ Measles | ✳ Lyme disease |

FIGURE 3-1 Infectious versus communicable disease.

from an invasion of a host from a disease-producing organism. This organism may be in the form of a virus, bacteria, fungus, or parasite. A **communicable disease** is an infectious disease that may be transmitted from one person to another. Employees at risk of occupational exposure to blood and body fluids should be especially concerned with human immunodeficiency virus (HIV), hepatitis B virus (HBV), hepatitis C virus (HCV), and tuberculosis (TB).

# DIRECT AND INDIRECT EXPOSURE

Exposure to communicable disease may occur by direct person-to-person contact through events such as sexual contact or a contaminated needlestick. Exposure may also be indirect through handling soiled linens or touching a contaminated object.

# CAUSES OF DISEASE

Although health care providers are often concerned with viral and bacterial diseases, one should realize that there are a number of other causes of infectious disease (Figure 3-2). Fungi, protozoa, and rickettsia are all

| Cause | Examples |
| --- | --- |
| Virus | Influenza, HIV, HBV |
| Bacteria | Tetanus, syphilis, tuberculosis |
| Helminth | Pinworms, tapeworms |
| Fungus | Tinea, dhobie itch |
| Protozoa | Malaria, dysentery |
| Rickettsia | Rocky Mountain spotted fever, typhus |

**FIGURE 3-2** Causes of infectious disease.

known to cause infectious disease. Descriptions of each of the main causes of infectious disease follow.

**Bacteria** are living microorganisms that can produce disease in a host. Bacteria can self-reproduce, and some may produce toxins that are harmful to their host. Bacteria are also capable of living outside the host. Diseases such as bacterial meningitis, tetanus, food poisoning, tuberculosis, and syphilis are caused by bacteria.

**Viruses** are microorganisms that reside within other living cells and cannot reproduce outside a living cell. Viruses such as HIV, HBV, HCV, and influenza may pose risks to those with occupational exposure.

**A fungus** is a plantlike organism that grows as single cells (e.g., yeast) or as multicellular colonies (e.g., mold). Since fungi do not contain chlorophyll, they depend on a **parasitic** or **saprophytic** existence. Examples of fungal infectious diseases include tinea (ringworm) and dhobie itch.

**Protozoans** are the simplest organisms in the animal kingdom. Many are single-celled, although some colonize. Examples of protozoal infections include malaria, dysentery, and sleeping sickness.

**Rickettsiae** are parasitic creatures who depend on living cells for growth. Usually transmitted by fleas, ticks, lice, and mites, infectious diseases caused by rickettsiae include Rocky Mountain spotted fever and several forms of typhus.

**Helminths** (worms) may also cause infectious disease. Although many worms are not parasitic, parasitic worms such as pinworms and tapeworms may be acquired by eating undercooked meat.

## INTERESTING FACTS

- ⊙ Malaria, a vector-borne disease carried primarily by mosquitoes, is both preventable and treatable. However, it kills approximately 1.2 million people each year, many of them young children in Africa. The United States reported 8 deaths in 2002.
- ⊙ While infectious diseases such as anthrax, botulism, and salmonellosis are not transmitted person-to-person, they may be used as weapons to affect large groups. (See Chapter 5 for more information.)
- ⊙ Ebola hemorrhagic fever (EHF) is considered one of the most virulent viral diseases known, causing death in 50 to 90% of cases.
- ⊙ Avian influenza (bird flu) was first discovered in Italy more than 100 years ago.
- ⊙ Bacteria are single-celled, but very complex.
- ⊙ Sick building syndrome is frequently caused by fungi.

# TRANSMISSION

When a communicable disease is passed from one person to another, a series of events takes place, creating a chain of infection (Figure 3-3). The first of these events is transmission, which may be airborne, bloodborne, or vector borne.

**Airborne transmission** is typically accomplished through droplets in a sneeze or cough. These aerosolized droplets travel through the air and are inhaled through the respiratory system or absorbed through mucous membranes. Tuberculosis is a common airborne transmissible disease.

### ALERT

It may be difficult to determine exposure to airborne transmissible disease. Health care providers should observe standard precautions when caring for any patient with a cough or sneezing.

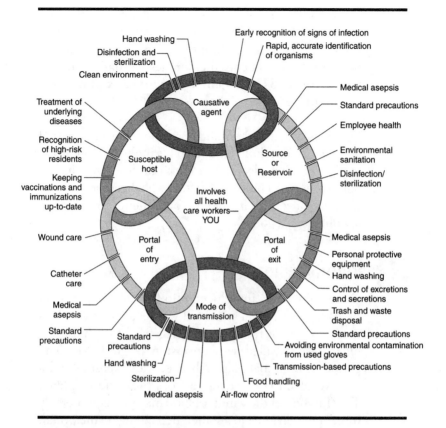

**FIGURE 3-3** Chain of infection. As with any chain, if one link is broken, the infection cannot be spread. This figure shows ways health care providers can break each link in the chain of infection.

**Bloodborne transmission** takes place when infected blood or blood-containing body fluid is introduced into the body of another person. Common ways this is accomplished are through needlesticks, splashing into the mucous membranes, or blood contacting nonintact skin.

**Vector-borne transmission** is transmission of a disease-causing organism through an outside source, or a vector. This includes a mosquito that carries malaria or a tick that carries Rocky Mountain spotted fever.

**Sexual transmission** is transmission of a disease through sexual contact with an infected person. Transmission is usually accomplished through the contact of infected body fluids with mucous membranes. **Sexually transmitted diseases (STDs)** include gonorrhea, syphilis, and genital herpes.

Some diseases are transmitted person-to-person by **casual contact** or **household contact.** This includes close body-to-body contact, sleeping in the same bed, and sharing hairbrushes or combs. Children who become infested with lice or scabies frequently catch them through casual contact at school.

# SEROCONVERSION

Once a disease is introduced into the body, a period of time elapses before a blood test will read "positive." This process of converting from a "negative" to a "positive" blood test is called **seroconversion** (Figure 3-4). The period of time that elapses between an exposure and a positive blood test is referred to as the **window phase.** The duration of the window phase may vary considerably from one individual to another, depending on the overall health, response of the immune system in the infected person, and the strength of the pathogen.

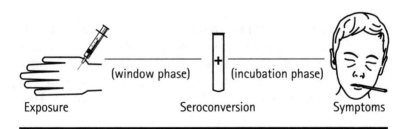

**FIGURE 3-4** Seroconversion progression. This figure illustrates the relationship of exposure to seroconversion and the appearance of the first symptoms.

# NEWSMAKER
## 25 Dead in 6 Days

PHILADELPHIA, PA                                                    JULY 30, 1976

To date, 25 people who attended the 58th annual American Legion state convention in philadelphia last week have died of a mysterious illness. Many more remain hospitalized in serious condition. Approximately 4400 people attended the convention.

The illnesses began as conventioneers began to return home from the July 21–24 gathering at the Bellevue-Stratford Hotel in Philadelphia's Center City. But now, American Legion members all across the state are becoming ill. At first, symptoms mimic those of the flu, including headache, fever, and general weakness. Then symptoms turn more severe—very much like pneumonia—including high fever, difficulty breathing, and chills.

At a news conference, Pennsylvania public health officials reported that autopsies on four of the dead revealed the cause of death to be severe viral pneumonia. Both the Pennsylvania Department of Public Health and the Centers for Disease Control continue to investigate the deaths and illness.

Postscript—In the days and weeks that followed, 34 convention participants died and 221 became ill. The common factor among them all was that they had all spent time at the Bellevue-Stratford Hotel, which closed shortly after the outbreak, but reopened in 1979. Without a name to give the mysterious disease, it took on an identity linked to those it affected most and became known as Legionnaires' disease. The rod-shaped bacterium that causes the disease was identified in January of the following year by CDC researchers and named *Legionella pneumophila*.

According to the survivors, the disease took its toll not only physically, but also mentally. Some Legionnaires recall that people avoided them, thinking that they might be contagious. "When I went in stores," said one member "they didn't want to touch my money."

It was never discovered exactly how the bacteria spread to infect the conventioneers. However, it was determined that although the Philadelphia outbreak is the most famous, it was not the first and certainly not the last outbreak of Legionnaires' disease. Researchers have learned that the *Legionella* bacterium was also responsible for causing the illness of 11 members who attended an Odd Fellows convention at the same hotel in 1974.

**UNDER THE MICROSCOPE**

❧ Research other outbreaks of Legionnaires' disease. Where have other outbreaks taken place? What type of environmental conditions seem to be amenable to the spread of *Legionella* bacterium?

❧ Search the Internet to learn the stories of some of those affected by the Philadelphia outbreak. Discuss these stories with your classmates.

Symptoms do not normally appear immediately with seroconversion. The time that passes between seroconversion and the appearance of symptoms is called the **incubation period.** For hepatitis B (HBV) this period may be up to 200 days. The incubation period for human immunodeficiency virus (HIV) may be as long as 10 years. Refer to Figure 3-5 for a summary of the possible stages of infectious disease.

It is important that both the patient and the caregiver realize that a single negative blood test and lack of immediate symptoms do not necessarily mean that a person is free from a disease. Follow-up testing at prescribed intervals is highly recommended.

The importance of protecting oneself from exposure to blood and **other potentially infectious material (OPIM)** is apparent when we realize that the carrier of HIV may display no signs or symptoms for up to 10 years.

Consider this example of why knowledge of seroconversion is important to health care providers.

Nancy, a registered nurse, is attending her son's Little League baseball game when another child is struck in the face by a batted ball, resulting in profuse bleeding from the nose and mouth. The patient appears in good health, but Nancy has no

| Latent period | Period after infection when an infectious agent cannot be transmitted to another host |
|---|---|
| Communicable period | Period after infection when an infectious agent can be transmitted to another host |
| Incubation period | Time between exposure and onset of symptoms |
| Window phase | Period during which antigen is present but seroconversion has not yet taken place |
| Disease period | Time between onset of symptoms and resolution of symptoms |

**FIGURE 3-5** Stages of infectious disease.

gloves readily available. She helps control the bleeding without the benefit of personal protective equipment (PPE). Although the child's young age and apparent state of health may make Nancy feel comfortable treating him without personal protective equipment, she may be placing herself in danger by assuming that he is free from infectious disease.

Suppose the seven-year-old has been exposed to hepatitis C (HCV) but does not yet know he is infected. Although he feels fine and looks healthy, he could still pass the virus on to anyone who comes in contact with his blood, including Nancy.

The point of this example is to show that regardless of how safe the patient looks, he may still be infected with a communicable disease.

### ALERT

Regardless of the situation, use standard precautions with every patient.

## CONCLUSION

By knowing how the disease process works, the employee at risk of occupational exposure can be better protected against exposure to disease.

## QUESTIONS FOR DISCUSSION

1. Are all infectious diseases communicable? Explain your answer.
2. Is a person more likely to become infected with HIV through direct or indirect contact? Explain your answer.
3. If you are exposed to blood or body fluids of a person with HIV today and have a negative blood test tomorrow, are you considered "safe"?
4. Name at least three ways diseases may be transmitted.
5. List at least four causes of infectious disease.

## WORTH THINKING ABOUT

- Which communicable disease(s) are you personally, as a health care provider, the most concerned with?
- Look at each link in the chain of infection and consider ways in which that link may be broken.

## WEB RESOURCES

**Legionnaires' disease** — This privately operated site provides a wealth of information about the history of Legionnaires' disease, including photos of and quotes from those who survived the 1976 Philadelphia outbreak. Visit this site at http://www.q-net.net.au/~legion.

**Journal of the American Medical Association** — For years, JAMA has been one of the leading journals for the medical profession. Visit the site at http://jama.ama-assn.org.

# BIBLIOGRAPHY

Centers for Disease Control and Prevention. (2000, April 21). *Escherichia coli* O111:H8 outbreak among teenage campers—Texas, 1999. *Morbidity and Mortality Weekly Report, 49* (15).

Green, D. (2005). *Legionnaires' disease: The first recorded outbreak.* http://q-net.net.au/~legion.

Neighbors, M., & Tannehill-Jones, R. (2000). *Human diseases.* Clifton Park, NY: Thomson Delmar Learning.

Shimeld, L. A., & Rodgers, A. T. (1999). *Essentials of diagnostic microbiology.* Clifton Park, NY: Thomson Delmar Learning.

Sugar, A. M., & Lyman, C. A. (1997). *A practical guide to medically important fungi and the diseases they cause.* Philadelphia: Lippincott-Raven.

Thibodeau, G. A., & Patton, K. T. (1999). *Anatomy and physiology.* (4th ed.). St. Louis: Mosby.

U. S. Fire Administration. (1992). *Guide to developing and managing an emergency service infection control program.* Emmitsburg, MD: U.S. Fire Administration.

# CHAPTER 4

# The Immune System

## LEARNING OBJECTIVES

After completing this chapter, the reader should be able to:

- describe the function and characteristics of the immune system.
- describe the body's defense mechanisms against infections.
- discuss and review anatomy and physiology related to the immune system.
- discuss the process of immune system defenses, including humoral and cell-mediated immunity.

## KEY TERMS

- acquired immunity
- active immunity
- antibodies
- antigens
- autoimmune response
- B lymphocytes
- basophils
- cancerous
- cell-mediated immunity
- chemotaxis
- complement proteins
- helper T cells

44

- humoral immunity
- inflammatory response
- inherited immunity
- integumentary system
- interferon
- killer T cells
- leukocytes
- lymphocytes
- lymphotoxin
- lysozyme
- macrophages
- mast cells
- mitotic
- natural killer cells
- neutrophils
- passive immunity
- phagocytosis
- sebum
- specific immunity
- T lymphocytes
- T suppressor cells
- therapeutic
- tumor

# INTRODUCTION

Every minute of every day, the immune system works to protect the body from pathogens. This chapter is intended to develop a basic understanding of the body's ability to protect itself and what one should expect when this system fails.

**FEATURED  CASE  STUDY**

Date:          June 23, 2005
Patient:       Mr. Charles Locke
Physician:     Dr. James Jeremiah

Mr. Locke is a 73-year-old male who presents to his doctor's office with hot reddened skin and itching and swelling on his right leg. He states that he scratched his leg on a piece of wire while bicycling. He is experiencing intermittent chills and has a temperature of 102.4°F. Pertinent medical history includes diabetes mellitus, type 1. Pus is oozing from the injured area.

1. What was the body's first line of defense against this infection? How was this defense breached?
2. What signs and symptoms consistent with infection are exhibited in this patient?
3. Explain why pus is present.
4. Could this infection have been prevented or at least its severity minimized? How?
5. What preexisting conditions might complicate this patient's current condition?
6. Are there other factors that might complicate this patient's current condition?

# STRUCTURE OF THE IMMUNE SYSTEM

The immune system is unique in that its components are not contained within one particular organ or organ system. The immune system is comprised of organs and structures from several other body systems, which work together to protect the body from pathogens. Some of the

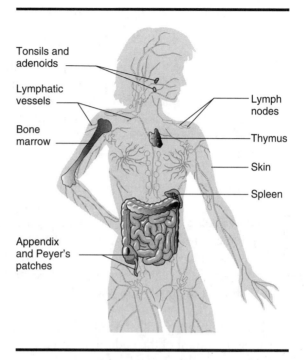

**FIGURE 4-1** Anatomy of the immune system.

major structures involved in immunity are discussed and are illustrated in Figure 4-1.

The tonsils form a protective ring around the upper throat and nose. The palatine tonsils are located on each side of the throat. The lingual tonsils are located near the base of the tongue. The pharyngeal tonsils (sometimes referred to as adenoids) are located near the posterior opening of the nasal cavity. Together, these lymphatic structures protect the entrance of the respiratory system against invading pathogens.

Lymph nodes are small oval or bean-shaped structures that range in size from a pin head to a lima bean. Lymph nodes are designed to filter harmful substances, including viruses, bacteria, and malignant cells.

Lymphatic vessels, which carry lymph from the tissues to the bloodstream, are very similar in structure to blood vessels, except that they are thinner and contain more valves to prevent backward flow of lymph fluid. Another difference is that lymphatic vessels contain lymph nodes at particular intervals.

The thymus is considered the primary organ of the lymphatic system. Located just above (superior to) the heart and just below (inferior to) the thyroid gland, the thymus produces T lymphocytes. As the final site of lymphocyte development before birth, the thymus is relatively large in infants. As we age, the thymus shrinks to the point at which little thymus tissue is found in adults.

The spleen is an oval-shaped organ located in the left upper quadrant of the abdomen, just above the left kidney, that serves several functions in the immune system. It is within the spleen that specialized white blood cells called monocytes and lymphocytes complete their development and are activated. The spleen also filters microorganisms and other foreign material from the blood through the process of phagocytosis. In addition, the spleen serves as a reservoir for blood that may be used when needed to destroy worn-out platelets and red blood cells and salvage the reusable components.

The vermiform appendix is a worm-like tube of lymphatic tissue that hangs from the lower portion of the cecum in the large intestine. The appendix serves as what could be described as a breeding ground for intestinal bacteria. Its function is not clear, but it is thought that the purpose of the appendix is to harbor nonpathogenic bacteria under normal conditions, which helps prevent disease. Peyer's patches are areas of lymphatic tissue located on the walls of the large intestine. They respond to antigens in the intestines by producing plasma cells that secrete antibodies.

The skin is an important part of the immune system. As a natural barrier against foreign pathogens, the skin protects the entire body from invasion. Bone marrow also works with the immune system and is important in the development of erythrocytes and leukocytes. Through the contributions of several body systems and organs working in concert with one another, the body is uniquely able to protect itself from most harmful pathogens.

# FUNCTION OF THE IMMUNE SYSTEM

The immune system protects the body from both external and internal assaults. When harmful microorganisms such as viruses, bacteria, or protozoans are introduced into the body, the immune system immediately springs into action to fight against these external assaults. Assaults may also be internal. When abnormal cells replicate and develop **tumors**, or new growths of tissue in which cell multiplication is uncontrolled, the immune system recognizes them as foreign and works to destroy them before they become **cancerous**, or capable of destructive growth and spread. Regardless of the source of the pathogen, the immune system constantly works to protect the body from foreign cells.

Sometimes foreign tissues are introduced into the body for **therapeutic** reasons. Organ and tissue transplants are sometimes recognized as foreign by the immune system and are rejected by the body. Occasionally the immune system will erroneously react to any part of the body that it

| Disease | Affected Area |
|---|---|
| Crohn's disease | Intestines, the ileum, or the colon |
| Diabetes mellitus, type 1 | Insulin-producing pancreatic cells |
| Graves' disease | Thyroid gland |
| Hashimoto's thyroiditis | Thyroid gland |
| Lupus erythematosus | Skin and other body systems |
| Myasthenia gravis | Nerve/muscle synapses |
| Multiple sclerosis | Brain and spinal cord |
| Psoriasis | Skin |
| Rheumatoid arthritis | Connective tissue |
| Scleroderma | Skin and other tissues |

**FIGURE 4-2** Examples of autoimmune disorders and the body systems they affect.

perceives as foreign. This elicits an **autoimmune response** and may result in illness. Examples of autoimmune disease include lupus, rheumatic fever, multiple sclerosis, and Graves' disease (Figure 4-2).

# THE IMMUNE RESPONSE

When pathogens enter the body, the immune system responds. Immunity typically falls into one of two categories. **Specific immunity** uses **lymphocytes** (T cells and B cells) to provide protection against specific pathogens. Nonspecific immunity uses neutrophils, macrophages, monocytes, and natural killer cells as a more general defense against pathogens. A description of each type of immunity follows.

# NEWSMAKER
## CBS Anchor Dead

NEW YORK, NY                                                    JULY 4, 1997

CBS Sunday Morning Anchor Kuralt Dead at Age 62

Charles Kuralt, CBS News' master storyteller, died today at New York Hospital from complications of lupus, an autoimmune disease that affects the skin, joints, kidneys, and nervous system. He was 62 years old.

Perhaps best known for his signature "On The Road" reports, Kuralt worked for CBS for 37 years as a reporter and anchorman. While reporting for CBS, Kuralt logged up to 50,000 miles per year on his motor home.

A native North Carolinian, Kuralt seemed to have a knack for finding great human interest stories and reported them in a way that touched his viewers. "All good television is about telling stories," said 60 Minutes executive producer Don Hewitt. "Nobody told them better than Charles Kuralt."

1. Charles Kuralt died of complications of lupus. What types of complications might you expect in a patient who has lupus?

2. Did Charles Kuralt fit the typical profile of a patient with lupus?

3. Name some common symptoms of lupus.

## UNDER THE MICROSCOPE

- Interview someone you know who has an autoimmune disease. Seek to discover the obstacles they face on a daily basis.
- Search the literature to learn about other famous people who have (or had) an autoimmune disease. See if you can find some famous animals affected by autoimmune disease.

# NONSPECIFIC IMMUNITY

The **integumentary system** provides the first line of defense against invasion by providing a structural barrier that prevents pathogens from readily entering the body. The skin also excretes **sebum** and perspiration, which mechanically wash pathogens off the skin and chemically attack bacteria. **Lysozyme**, an enzyme that attacks cell walls of gram-positive bacteria, causes skin to be acidotic, making it inhospitable to most bacteria. The skin constantly regenerates itself by sloughing off the old layer along with external irritants.

The respiratory system provides protection against inhaled irritants. Coughs and sneezes help remove pathogens from the upper airway, and mucus and cilia within the respiratory tract help to trap and mechanically remove irritants. The structure of the tonsils also protects the entrance of the respiratory system from invading pathogens.

Gastric acids and enzymes also help neutralize pathogens that attack through the gastrointestinal system. The presence of normal bacterial flora may also produce chemicals that inhibit the growth of invading bacteria.

Dangerous pathogens may also be removed from the body via mechanical methods. Pathogens are sloughed off with dead skin cells, vomited from the stomach, flushed from the urinary tract with urine, or caught in respiratory mucus and coughed up. Both the anatomic structure and the mechanical function of the body serve as first-line defense against invasion by harmful pathogens.

# INFLAMMATORY RESPONSE

If anatomic barriers like the skin form the first line of protection against pathogens, the inflammatory response provides the second line of protection. The **inflammatory**

**response** uses specialized leukocytes called neutrophils and macrophages to find and destroy invading pathogens through a process called phagocytosis.

When an injury or invasion takes place, **leukocytes,** or white blood cells, are summoned to the affected area through a release of leukocyte-attracting chemicals in a process called **chemotaxis**. This results in increased blood flow and vascular permeability in the area, causing the characteristic signs of infection, including hot, swollen, and reddened skin (Figure 4-3).

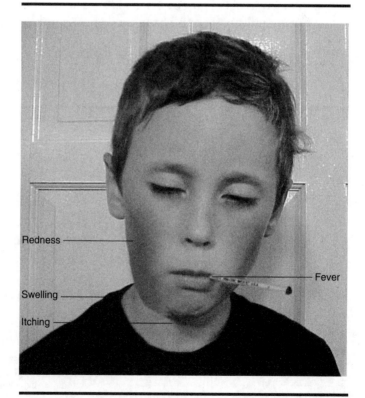

**FIGURE 4-3** Health care providers should be alert to the signs and symptoms of infection, including reddened skin, fever, swelling, and itching.

## Phagocytosis

Another part of the inflammatory process is **phagocytosis**. In this process, phagocytes (cells capable of phagocytosis) attack and ingest the invading agent. Phagocytes attack invading pathogens by trapping them with an arm-like projection and encircling them by forming a sac around them. Once enclosed in a sac, the pathogens are chemically destroyed.

Two of the most common phagocytes are **neutrophils** and **macrophages** (Figure 4-4). Neutrophils are the most numerous of the phagocytes. Soon after injury or invasion, neutrophils come out of the capillaries into the affected area, where they ingest the microorganisms through phagocytosis and die within 1 or 2 days. Because of this short life

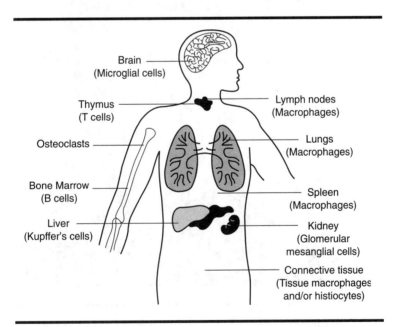

**FIGURE 4-4** Cells of the immune system. The immune system is made up of cells from many body systems.

span, dead neutrophils tend to aggregate and form pus, which is readily absorbed into the surrounding tissues.

Macrophages migrate out of the bloodstream and grow to several times their original size. They may reside on the surface of mucous membranes for long periods of time. Frequently found in the alveoli, lymph nodes, brain, liver, and spleen, macrophages ingest invading and dead cells. Like neutrophils, dead macrophages tend to collect in the affected area as pus.

## Other Types of Nonspecific Immunity

Other types of nonspecific immunity include the following.

* **natural killer cells**—Natural killer cells are another type of lymphocyte that recognizes and destroys infectious or tumor cells. Natural killer cells do not have to be activated by an external antigen, so they are considered nonspecific.
* **interferon**—Interferon is a protein that defends against viral infections. By inhibiting the ability of a virus to cause a disease, interferon prevents viruses from replicating in cells.
* **complement proteins**—A group of approximately 20 inactivated plasma proteins called complement, circulate in the blood. When activated, complement proteins cause rupture of the cell that triggered them. Complement proteins may be triggered by both specific and nonspecific mechanisms.

## S PECIFIC IMMUNITY

Specific immunity allows the body to defend against specific foreign pathogens within the body. Specific immunity may be either acquired or inherited. **Inherited immunity** is, as the name implies, obtained in utero.

**Acquired immunity** may be natural, resulting from non-deliberate exposure to antigens after birth; or artificial, brought about by immunization.

## Active and Passive Immunity

Acquired immunity, whether natural or artificial, may be active or passive. **Active immunity** means that the individual has the ability to produce antibodies to a certain antigen. This type of immunity is longer acting than passive immunity.

**Passive immunity** refers to immunity that is from an outside source or transferred to someone who was not previously immune. Passive immunity provides temporary, but immediate, protection.

# COMPONENTS OF SPECIFIC IMMUNITY

As with nonspecific immunity, several components work together to protect the body from invasion from specific pathogens. Descriptions of some of the more important ones follow.

## Antigens and Antibodies

**Antigens** are chemical markers that identify cells as self (human) or nonself (foreign). When viruses, bacteria, or fungi are recognized as foreign, they are marked as nonself by antigens and subsequently destroyed by the immune system.

**Antibodies** work in a similar fashion, although they are much more specific. Produced in plasma, antibodies are proteins that attach themselves to antigens to mark them for destruction. Each antibody is specific to only one antigen, and the body may produce millions of different antibodies when needed. The five major classes of antibodies follow.

- *Immunoglobulin A (IgA)* is found primarily in the mucous membranes, saliva, and tears. Among other things, it provides passive immunity for breast-fed infants and combines with a protein in the mucosa to defend against invading microorganisms.
- *Immunoglobulin D (IgD)* is found in the B lymphocytes and accounts for less than 1% of antibodies. Its exact function is not known.
- *Immunoglobulin E (IgE)* is found in the **mast cells** or **basophils,** and accounts for less than 1% of antibodies. It is important to the immediate histamine response in allergic reactions.
- *Immunoglobulin G (IgG)* is the most abundant circulating antibody, and is located in the blood and extracellular fluid. IgG has four subclasses and deals primarily with the secondary immune response. It also has the distinction of being the only immunoglobulin that has the ability to cross the placenta to provide temporary immunity in neonates.
- *Immunoglobulin M (IgM)* is the dominant antibody responsible for the primary immune response. IgM also increases production of IgG in acute infections.

## B Lymphocytes

**B lymphocytes** (B cells) develop in two stages. Inactive B cells develop by the time an infant reaches a few months of age, and make antibody molecules that attach to the surface of plasma membranes, serving as receptors for specific antigens. After being released from the bone marrow, inactive B cells find their way to the lymph nodes and spleen.

When a B cell comes in contact with the specific antigen that activates it, the antibodies on the B cell's surface bind to the antigen. This triggers a series of **mitotic** divisions. As this rapid division takes place, the B cell produces a set of clones. Some of these clones form plasma cells, which make and secrete large amounts of antibody.

Other clones stay in the lymphatic tissue as memory cells. Should the clone come in contact with the antigen again, memory cells can become plasma cells, which can secrete antibodies, protecting the body from a previously encountered antigen.

 **INTERESTING FACTS**

- Over 8.5 million Americans had autoimmune diseases in 1996.
- According to the Lupus Foundation of America, more than half of those afflicted with lupus suffered for 4 years or more before being diagnosed.
- Females are nine times more likely to contract lupus than are males.
- 75% of cases of autoimmune disease occur in women.

## Humoral Immunity

Since B cells do not destroy pathogens directly, but instead produce antibodies that destroy a specific antigen, the process of immunity they produce is called *antibody-mediated immunity*. It is also called **humoral immunity** because it occurs within plasma, which is one of the humors (fluids) in the body.

## T Lymphocytes

**T lymphocytes,** or T cells, attack pathogens directly. The immunity they provide is sometimes referred to as **cell-mediated immunity**. T cells are lymphocytes that develop in the thymus and typically reside in the spleen and lymph nodes. There are three types of T cells.

- **Killer T cells** are able to recognize, bind to, and kill antigens located on the surface of pathogenic cells. By releasing **lymphotoxin,** a powerful poison, T killer cells eliminate pathogens directly.

- **Helper T cells** work with **T suppressor cells** to regulate the function of B cells and other T cells.

## Cell-Mediated Immunity

Since T cells directly locate and destroy diseased or pathogenic cells, the type of immunity offered by T cells is referred to as *cell-mediated immunity*. The cells themselves defend the body against dangerous pathogens.

## CONCLUSION

The human body is capable of defending itself against pathogens, both internal and external. The combination of nonspecific and specific immunity ensures maximum protection against any pathogen, foreign cell, or cancerous tumor. It is important for health care professionals to understand the fundamentals of the immune system so they can recognize signs that would indicate when the immune system is reacting to a pathogen.

## QUESTIONS FOR DISCUSSION

1. List and describe some of the key anatomical structures of the immune system.
2. Describe the process of phagocytosis and explain why it results in the production of pus.
3. Which lasts longer, passive or active immunity? Why?
4. Of antigens and antibodies, which are more specific? Why?
5. List several signs and symptoms of infections. Discuss why these signs appear.

## WORTH THINKING ABOUT

- Think of a time when you had an infection. Recall the signs and symptoms you exhibited. What evidence did this give you of your immune system at work?

## WEB RESOURCES

**How Stuff Works**—This innovative site is an excellent resource for information on a variety of topics, including immunity. Visit the site at http://www.howstuffworks.com.

**National Cancer Institute**—This National Institutes of Health site provides information and data on cancer and cancer research. Subscribe to the NCI bulletin. Visit the site at http://www.cancer.gov.

**Medline Plus**—This U.S. National Library of Medicine and National Institutes of Health site provides a great deal of health information, including information on autoimmune diseases and cancer. http://medlineplus.gov.

## BIBLIOGRAPHY

Cable News Network (1997, July 4). Charles Kuralt, CBS' poet of small-town America, dies at 62. http://www.cnn.com.

Cure Research (2005). http://www.cureresearch.com.

Hegner, B. R., Caldwell, E., & Needham, J. F. (2004). *Nursing assistant: A nursing process approach.* (9th ed.). Clifton Park, NY: Thomson Delmar Learning.

Lupus Foundation of America (2005). http://www.lupus.org.

Neighbors, M., & Tannehill-Jones, R. (2000). *Human diseases.* Clifton Park, NY: Thomson Delmar Learning.

Pike, R. (2005, July 5). Road ends for Charles Kuralt. South Coast Today. http://www.s-t.com.

Smith, J. (1995). *Immunology: The clinical laboratory manual series.* Clifton Park, NY: Thomson Delmar Learning.

Thibodeau, G. A., & Patton, K. T. (1999). *Anatomy and physiology.* (4th ed.). St. Louis: Mosby.

Van Wynsberghe, D., Noback, C. R., & Carola, R. (1995). *Human anatomy and physiology.* (3rd ed.). New York: McGraw-Hill.

## CHAPTER 5

# Protection from Communicable Disease in the Workplace

## LEARNING OBJECTIVES

After completing this chapter, the reader should be able to:

- list and describe common engineering controls and work practices.
- discuss the importance of personal health to the health care provider.
- discuss the risks, benefits, and side effects of the hepatitis B vaccine.
- list the vaccines recommended for health care providers by the CDC.
- discuss the proper disposal of contaminated supplies.
- demonstrate the cleaning and disinfection of patient care areas.
- demonstrate the cleaning and disinfection of patient care equipment.
- demonstrate proper use of personal protective equipment.
- demonstrate proper hand washing technique.
- list the three levels of the Spaulding Classification System.
- explain the difference between cleaning, disinfecting, and sterilizing.
- define health care–associated and nosocomial infections.

- list and describe three sources of nosocomial infections.
- list strategies to prevent nosocomial infections.

## KEY TERMS

- airborne precautions
- biohazard container
- body substance isolation (BSI)
- cleaning
- contact precautions
- critical
- cross-contamination
- disinfection
- droplet precautions
- endogenous flora
- engineering controls
- essential functions
- exogenous flora
- fit-tested
- health care–associated infection (HAI)
- National Institute for Occupational Safety & Health (NIOSH)
- NIOSH-approved respirator
- noncritical
- nosocomial infections
- particulate respirator
- personal health
- personal protective equipment (PPE)
- pre-entry physical exam
- safe work practices
- sharps containers
- semicritical
- Spaulding Classification System

- spores
- standard precautions
- sterilization
- transmission-based precautions
- universal biohazard symbol

## FEATURED CASE STUDY

Date:        June 19, 1994
Patient:     Elise Falco
Paramedic:   Waldo Witherspoon

While enjoying a relaxing weekend off, Waldo Witherspoon, a paramedic working for a small rural ambulance service received a call from central dispatch. A serious motor vehicle collision had occurred in his community. An ambulance had been dispatched, but because of the nature of the call, it was expected that additional help would be needed. The dispatcher asked Witherspoon to respond in his personal vehicle to assist the crew.

Upon arrival, Witherspoon found that a military Humvee® had crashed head on into a sedan occupied by two elderly females. The ambulance was on the scene and the paramedic had called for a medical helicopter to transport both patients, including Ms. Elise Falco. Witherspoon was asked to attend to Ms. Falco while the other paramedic took care of another patient.

As he climbed in the back of the ambulance, an EMT handed Witherspoon a pair of gloves. As Witherspoon was donning gloves, the EMT quickly applied an antishock garment to the patient. Witherspoon worked quickly to assess the patient, start intravenous lines, and ensure that the patient was ready for helicopter transport.

When the helicopter arrived, Witherspoon assisted with loading the patients, then retreated behind the ambulance while the craft took off. As the ambulance crew thanked him for his help one of them noticed a splatter of blood on Witherspoon's face and neck. Judging from the pattern on the right side of his face, it appeared likely that some blood had been splattered in his right eye.

1. What could have prevented this occupational potential exposure to blood?
2. When should personal protective equipment (PPE) be used?
3. What vaccinations should Witherspoon have had that would help protect him from communicable disease?

# INTRODUCTION

Protection from communicable disease is a joint responsibility of the employer and the employee. This chapter addresses the responsibilities of each and how the employer and employee must work together to achieve optimal protection.

# ENGINEERING CONTROLS

Engineering controls are actions taken by the employer to make the workplace safer by engineering safety directly into the workplace. This may include anything from placement of sharps containers and hand washing facilities to providing adequate storage facilities for hazardous chemicals. This may entail making the surfaces of work areas easy to clean and sanitize, or installing adequate air handling and ventilation equipment. In short, engineering controls make safe practices practical and convenient for the employee.

## Hand Washing Facilities

Hand washing facilities, including hot water, soap, and a mechanism for drying should be made available and accessible to all health care providers. When traditional hand washing is impractical, alcohol-based cleaner should be made available.

## Alcohol Hand Cleaners

The Centers for Disease Control and Prevention (CDC) guidelines recommend the use of alcohol-based agents for hand washing, especially in situations in which soap and running water are not readily available. These guidelines are based on scientific evidence and are consistent with the Bloodborne Pathogen standard of the Occupational Safety and Health Administration (OSHA).

Studies show that alcohol-based hand cleaners are effective, play a role in improving hand washing compliance, and result in a low incidence of dermatitis. For greatest effectiveness in killing germs, the U.S. Food and Drug Administration recommends a concentration of 60% to 95% alcohol. When using an alcohol-based cleaner, the product should be applied to the palm of one hand. Rub hands together until dry, ensuring that all hand and finger surfaces are covered.

## Biohazard Containers

The employer must also provide readily accessible **biohazard containers** for the disposal of contaminated materials. **Sharps containers** (Figure 5-1) are closable,

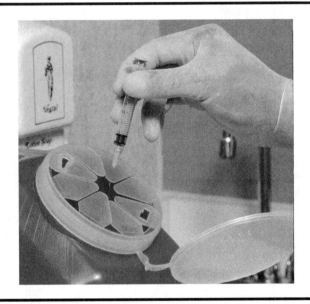

**FIGURE 5-1** Biohazard container used for proper disposal of sharp objects such as IV needles and sutures.

puncture-resistant containers used to dispose of contaminated needles, scalpels, sutures and other sharps, such as disposable razors and broken glass. OSHA's Bloodborne Pathogen standard requires these containers to be not only closable and puncture resistant, but also to be leakproof on the sides and bottom, and to be labeled or color coded in accordance with the standard.

OSHA also requires that sharps containers be:

- easily accessible and located near the area where sharps are used.
- maintained upright throughout use.
- replaced routinely and not be allowed to become overfilled.

When sharps containers are moved, OSHA requires that they be closed (to prevent spillage) and, if leakage is possible, placed in a secondary container that must be closable and constructed in such a way as to contain its contents and prevent leakage during handling or transport.

## Labeling

For biohazards other than sharps, a variety of containers may be used, as long they are labeled according to the following requirements:

* Warning labels shall be affixed to containers of regulated waste, refrigerators and freezers containing blood or other potentially infectious material, and other containers used to store, transport, or ship blood or other potentially infectious materials. Labels shall be fluorescent red or orange-red, with letters and symbols in a contrasting color.

* Labels shall be affixed as close as feasible to the container by string, wire, adhesive, or other method that prevents loss or unintentional removal.

When appropriate, bags (Figure 5-2) and other containers may be used as long as they display the **universal biohazard symbol** (Figure 5-3) or are red in color. Containers of blood, blood components, or blood products that are labeled as to their contents and have been released for transfusion or other clinical use are exempted from these labeling requirements.

## Medical Devices

In recent years medical device manufacturers have worked toward engineering safety directly into devices such as needles, syringes, and diagnostic equipment (Figure 5-4). Intravenous placement sets are now available, which offer extra protection by allowing the needle to be retracted into a secure container before being detached from the patient catheter. Some blood-drawing

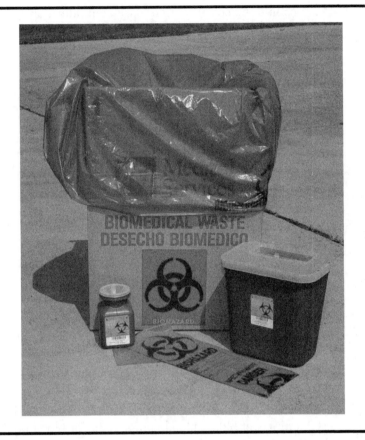

**FIGURE 5-2** Although the external container may vary, the presence of a red bag indicates that the contents are biohazardous.

needles have the feature of shielding the needle before it is withdrawn from the vein or artery. Syringes are being made with protective shields to cover the needle or with needles that retract into the barrel of the syringe after use.

According to the **National Institute for Occupational Safety and Health (NIOSH)**, protected-needle and needleless IV systems have decreased needlestick

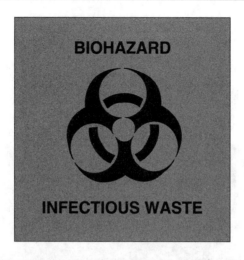

**FIGURE 5-3** The universal biohazard symbol has an orange or red background with a contrasting color symbol.

injuries caused by attaching a syringe to an IV connector by as much as 88%. Studies also show that phlebotomy (blood-drawing) injuries were reduced by 82% through the use of a needle shield.

Health care providers should remember that improved medical devices are engineered with safety in mind but are not a replacement for safe work practices or individuals taking care with their work.

## Other Concerns

Eye wash stations, when applicable, should be accessible and maintained in good working condition. Care should be taken to ensure that eye wash stations are placed in appropriate locations and that all employees understand how to operate them.

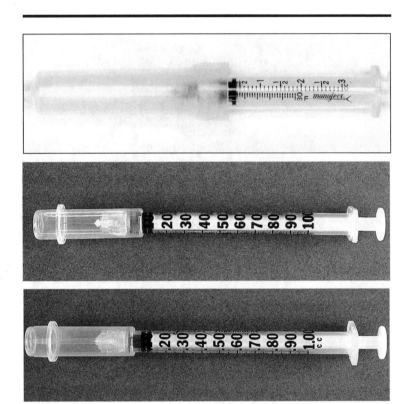

**FIGURE 5-4** Medical devices with built-in safety features.

When potentially hazardous chemicals (including many cleaning compounds) are used, they must be properly labeled and stored in appropriate locations near where they are used. Material Safety Data Sheets (MSDS), which give persons working with or responding to emergencies involving chemicals specific information on physical properties, toxicity, and first aid, must be available and accessible to those who use the chemicals in their work.

Engineering controls are considered the responsibility of the employer, but the employee is responsible for notifying the employer about engineering controls that are necessary to promote safe work practices.

# SAFE WORK PRACTICES

**Safe work practices** are typically considered a responsibility of the employee. The employer, however, is responsible for ensuring compliance with these practices. Safe work practices should be listed in the employer's standard operating procedure or employee handbook. Figure 5-5 shows examples of common safe work practices.

## Hand Washing

Hand washing is arguably the most important work practice and is cited by the Association for Professionals in Infection Control and Epidemiology as being the single most important work practice for preventing nosocomial infections. Figure 5-6 features a listing of hand washing tips.

Employees should be instructed in proper hand washing techniques and employers should ensure compliance with proper hand washing procedures. Employees should

---

- The employee must not eat or drink while in a work area.
- The employee must not smoke while in a work area.
- The employee must not handle contact lenses in a work area.
- The employee must not apply makeup or lip balm in a work area.
- The employee must wash hands after contact with each patient.
- The employee must wear appropriate protective equipment when providing patient care.

---

**FIGURE 5-5** Examples of safe work practices.

---

- Wash your hands. It is the single most important procedure for preventing nosocomial infections.
- Wash your hands after prolonged or intense contact with any patient.
- Wash your hands before and after situations where contamination is likely.
- Wash your hands after removing gloves.
- When in doubt, wash your hands.

---

**FIGURE 5-6** Hand washing tips. (*Source:* Association for Professionals in Infection Control and Epidemiology, Inc.)

wash their hands for at least 15 seconds with soap and running warm water before and after each contact with a patient and after removing gloves. One of the greatest problems with hand washing is that when improperly done, the employee's hands can be contaminated before the hand washing procedure is complete. Figure 5-7 outlines a suggested hand washing technique that will help prevent recontamination.

OSHA recognizes that some work areas, especially outside the hospital, may not have access to running water. In these cases, the employer must provide antiseptic towelettes or alcohol hand cleaner to accommodate hand washing.

### Handling and Using Sharps

Needles, sutures, and scalpels are common tools of the trade for many health care providers. Because of the possibility of injury and contamination through accidental cuts and sticks with these devices, health care providers should use extreme care when working with or disposing

## Proper Hand Washing Technique

To avoid recontamination during hand washing,
follow this procedure.

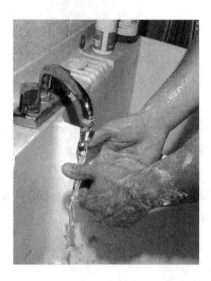

1. Make paper towel readily available. A common mistake is to wash hands and then access paper towels. This contaminates clean hands.
2. Turn water on.
3. Dispense soap. The use of liquid soap is preferred over bar soap.
4. Rub soaped hands vigorously under running water. Rinse from proximal to distal. (forearms to fingertips)
5. With the water still running, dry hands with previously dispensed towel. Use the towel to turn the water off. This will prevent you from contaminating your clean hands by touching the towel dispenser or the faucet handle.
6. Dispose of the towel in an appropriate container.

**FIGURE 5-7** Suggested hand washing procedure.

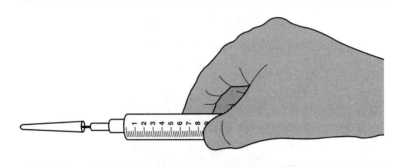

**FIGURE 5-8** One-handed technique to recap a needle. Although recapping is not recommended, use the one-handed technique when recapping is necessary.

of these items. Over 800,000 needlestick incidents occur each year in U.S. hospitals. Many of these incidents occur after the needle was used and approximately 1/3 occur during disposal.

As a general rule, needles should be disposed of immediately after use and should not be bent or recapped. If it is necessary to recap a needle, a one-handed technique should be used. Figure 5-8 illustrates a one-handed technique for recapping needles.

# ISOLATION PRACTICES

As early as 1877, health care providers used the principle of isolation to combat the spread of **nosocomial,** or **health care–associated, infections.** Then, patients with infectious diseases were isolated from noninfected patients in an effort to control the spread of infection within the hospital population. Today, facilities use a two-tiered system of precautions developed by the Centers for Disease Control and Prevention (CDC) with the same goal, but with more clearly defined guidelines.

## Standard and Transmission-Based Precautions

The first tier, **standard precautions**, is used with all patients, and advocates isolation from blood, nonintact skin, mucous membranes, and all body fluids with the exception of perspiration (Figure 5-9). **Transmission-based precautions**, the second tier, are used with patients known or suspected to be infected with highly transmissible or epidemiologically important pathogens. One or more of three types of transmission-based precautions may be used, depending on the way a given disease is transmitted.

## Airborne Precautions

**Airborne precautions** (Figure 5-10) are used for patients known or suspected to be infected with airborne transmissible diseases like tuberculosis and measles. Emphasis is placed on patient placement and respiratory protection. Patients should be isolated from other patients and placed in an area with negative-pressure ventilation. **A NIOSH-approved respirator** should be worn by all caregivers.

## Droplet Precautions

**Droplet precautions** (Figure 5-11) are used to protect the health care provider from inhaling large particle droplets of moisture that carry contaminants. The patient should be isolated from other patients when possible. Health care providers should wear masks when working within 3 feet of the patient.

## Contact Precautions

**Contact precautions** (Figure 5-12) deal with coming in contact with an infected person or their personal items, such as bed linens or clothing. The patient should be

**STANDARD PRECAUTIONS**
FOR INFECTION CONTROL

**Wash Hands** (Plain soap)
Wash after touching **blood, body fluids, secretions, excretions,** and **contaminated items.** Wash immediately **after gloves are removed** and **between patient contacts.** Avoid transfer of microorganisms to other patients or environments.

**Wear Gloves**
Wear when touching **blood, body fluids, secretions, excretions,** and **contaminated items.** Put on **clean** gloves just **before touching mucous membranes** and **nonintact skin.** Change gloves between tasks and procedures on the same patient after contact with material that may contain high concentrations of microorganisms. Remove gloves promptly after use, before touching noncontaminated items and environmental surfaces, and before going to another patient, and wash hands immediately to avoid transfer of microorganisms to other patients or environments.

**Wear Mask and Eye Protection or Face Shield**
Protect mucous membranes of the eyes, nose, and mouth during procedures and patient-care activities that are likely to generate **splashes** or **sprays** of **blood, body fluids, secretions,** or **excretions.**

**Wear Gown**
Protect skin and prevent soiling of clothing during procedures that are likely to generate **splashes** or **sprays** of **blood, body fluids, secretions,** or **excretions.** Remove a soiled gown as promptly as possible and wash hands to avoid transfer of microorganisms to other patients or environments.

**Patient-Care Equipment**
Handle used patient-care equipment soiled with **blood, body fluids, secretions,** or **excretions** in a manner that prevents skin and mucous membrane exposures, contamination of clothing, and transfer of microorganisms to other patients and environments. Ensure that reusable equipment is not used for the care of another patient until it has been appropriately cleaned and reprocessed and single use items are properly discarded.

**Environmental Control**
Follow hospital procedures for routine care, cleaning, and disinfection of environmental surfaces, beds, bed rails, bedside equipment, and other frequently touched surfaces.

**Linen**
Handle, transport, and process used linen soiled with **blood, body fluids, secretions,** or **excretions** in a manner that prevents exposures and contamination of clothing, and avoids transfer of microorganisms to other patients and environments.

**Occupational Health and Bloodborne Pathogens**
Prevent injuries when using needles, scalpels, and other sharp instruments or devices; when handling sharp instruments after procedures; when cleaning used instruments; and when disposing of used needles.

**Never recap used needles using both hands** or any other technique that involves directing the point of a needle toward any part of the body; rather, use either a one-handed "scoop" technique or a mechanical device designed for holding the needle sheath.

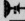

Do not remove used needles from disposable syringes by hand, and do not bend, break, or otherwise manipulate used needles by hand. Place used disposable syringes and needles, scalpel blades, and other sharp items in puncture-resistant sharps containers located as close as practical to the area in which the items were used, and place reusable syringes and needles in a puncture-resistant container for transport to the reprocessing area.

Use **resuscitation devices** as an alternative to mouth-to-mouth resuscitation.

**Patient Placement**
Use a **private room** for a patient who contaminates the environment or who does not (or cannot be expected to) assist in maintaining appropriate hygiene or environmental control. Consult Infection Control if a private room is not available.

**FIGURE 5-9** Standard precautions. *(Courtesy of BREVIS Corporation, Salt Lake City, UT)*

**AIRBORNE PRECAUTIONS**
**(in addition to Standard Precautions)**
**VISITORS: Report to nurse before entering.**

**Patient Placement**
Use **private room** that has:
   Monitored negative air pressure,
   6 to 12 air changes per hour,
   Discharge of air outdoors or HEPA filtration if
   recirculated.
**Keep room door closed and patient in room.**

**Respiratory Protection**
Wear an **N95 respirator** when entering the room of a
patient with known or suspected infectious pulmonary
**tuberculosis.**
**Susceptible** persons should not enter the room of
patients known or suspected to have **measles** (rubeola)
or **varicella** (chickenpox) if other immune caregivers are
available. If susceptible persons must enter, they should
wear an **N95 respirator.** (Respirator or surgical mask
not required if immune to measles and varicella.)

**Patient Transport**
Limit transport of patient from room to essential purposes
only. Use **surgical mask** on patient during transport.

**FIGURE 5-10** Airborne precautions. *(Courtesy of BREVIS Corporation, Salt Lake City, UT)*

isolated from other patients to the extent possible. Gloves
should be worn when caring for the patient and removed
immediately after patient contact. Hand washing with
soap and warm running water should take place after
removing gloves. When it is anticipated that the care
giver will have substantial contact with the patient or
his/her belongings, or when the patient is incontinent,
has diarrhea, an ileostomy, a colostomy, or drainage from
a wound not controlled by a dressing, a gown that is

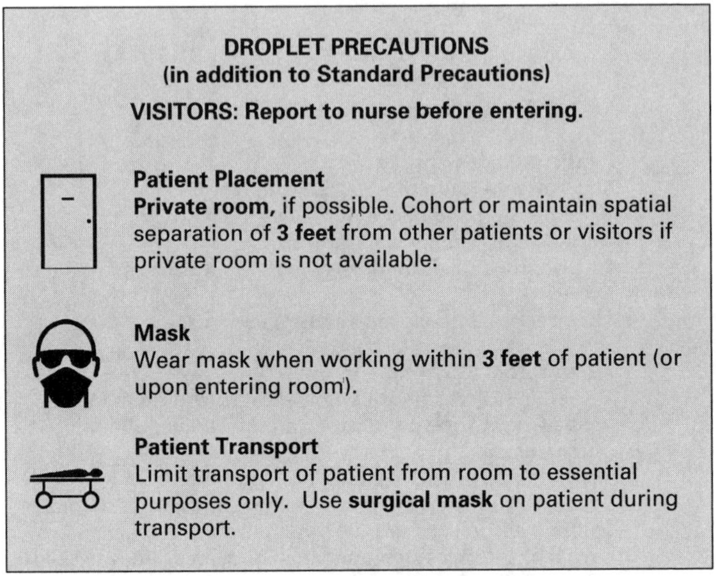

---

**DROPLET PRECAUTIONS**
**(in addition to Standard Precautions)**

**VISITORS: Report to nurse before entering.**

**Patient Placement**
**Private room,** if possible. Cohort or maintain spatial separation of **3 feet** from other patients or visitors if private room is not available.

**Mask**
Wear mask when working within **3 feet** of patient (or upon entering room).

**Patient Transport**
Limit transport of patient from room to essential purposes only. Use **surgical mask** on patient during transport.

---

**FIGURE 5-11** Droplet precautions. *(Courtesy of BREVIS Corporation, Salt Lake City, UT)*

impervious to liquid should be worn. The gown should be removed and disposed of after each patient contact. Keep exposure to other patients to a minimum and use care in ensuring that patient care equipment used with a patient on contact isolation is limited to use with only that patient.

# NOSOCOMIAL INFECTIONS

Nosocomial infections, sometimes called **health care–associated infections (HAIs)**, are infections that originate in a health care setting. In the United States, HAIs account for an estimated 2 million infections and 90,000 deaths annually.

---

**CONTACT PRECAUTIONS**
(in addition to Standard Precautions)
VISITORS: Report to nurse before entering.

**Patient Placement**
**Private room,** if possible. Cohort if private room is not available.

**Gloves**
Wear gloves when entering patient room.
**Change** gloves after having contact with infective material that may contain high concentrations of microorganisms **(fecal** material and **wound drainage). Remove** gloves before leaving patient room.

**Wash**
Wash hands with an **antimicrobial** agent immediately after glove removal. After glove removal and handwashing, ensure that hands do not touch potentially contaminated environmental surfaces or items in the patient's room to avoid transfer of microorganisms to other patients or environments.

**Gown**
Wear gown when entering patient room if you anticipate that your clothing will have a substantial contact with the patient, environmental surfaces, or items in the patient's room, or if the patient is **incontinent,** or has **diarrhea,** an **ileostomy, a colostomy,** or **wound drainage** not contained by a dressing. **Remove** gown before leaving the patient's environment and ensure that clothing does not contact potentially contaminated environmental surfaces to avoid transfer of microorganisms to other patients or environments.

**Patient Transport**
Limit transport of patient to essential purposes only. During transport, ensure that precautions are maintained to minimize the risk of transmission of microorganisms to other patients and contamination of environmental surfaces and equipment.

**Patient-Care Equipment**
Dedicate the use of noncritical patient-care equipment to a single patient. If common equipment is used, clean and disinfect between patients.

---

**FIGURE 5–12** Contact precautions. *(Courtesy of BREVIS Corporation, Salt Lake City, UT)*

Most nosocomial infections come from **endogenous flora,** that is, organisms from the patient's own body. Other sources include **exogenous flora** (the environment) and **cross-contamination** from staff and other patients.

Strategies to prevent nosocomial infections include:

- Adherence to infection control practices.
- Thorough hand washing before and after touching each patient.
- Careful attention to cleaning, disinfecting, and sterilizing patient-care equipment, supplies, and instruments.

# OUT-OF-HOSPITAL ISOLATION

**Body substance isolation (BSI)** contends that all body substances are infectious and employees must protect themselves from contact with any body substance. This system of protection is generally preferred by prehospital care providers, industrial responders, and employees in many emergency departments. Emphasis is on maximal, rather than minimal, protection.

# PERSONAL PROTECTIVE EQUIPMENT

**Personal protective equipment (PPE)** is provided by the employer for use by the employee for protection from exposure to contaminants in the workplace. Personal protective equipment must be readily available at the work site or issued to employees for use.

### ALERT

Gloves should be replaced after each patient contact.

## Gloves

Gloves are the most frequently used PPE. OSHA requires that employers provide each employee with gloves that fit properly. Persons with an allergy to latex must be provided with glove liners or nonallergenic, nonlatex gloves at no cost to the employee. Gloves should be discarded and replaced as soon as practical after becoming soiled. Remember, the use of gloves does not eliminate the need to wash hands properly. The employee should wash hands immediately after removing gloves.

## ALERT

People who wash their hands frequently and/or wear gloves often may need to use lotion to keep their hands from cracking, thereby creating a potential portal of entry for pathogens.

## Masks and Respirators

Face masks provide little protection against airborne transmissible diseases, but may be helpful as an adjunct to eye protection when there is a possibility of splashing blood or body fluids. There are times when it may be appropriate to apply a mask to a patient who is sneezing or coughing.

**Particulate respirators** protect the wearer by filtering out airborne particles. A variety of respirators, which must be approved by NIOSH, are available. Health care professionals may wear any NIOSH-approved respirator. Approved respirators will be marked with the NIOSH designation, the manufacturer's name, the part number (P/N), and the protection provided by the filter. Those who wear respirators must be medically screened for fitness to wear a respirator and must be **fit-tested** (Figure 5-13) for each device. A variety of respirators are shown in Figure 5-14.

Respirators should be selected based on the expected hazards. For instance, exposure to a patient with tuberculosis requires a respirator.

### Donning instructions (to be followed each time product is worn):

**1** Cup the respirator in your hand with the nosepiece at fingertips, allowing the headbands to hang freely below hands.

**2** Position the respirator under your chin with the nosepiece up.

**3** Pull the top strap over your head so it rests high on the back of head.

**4** Pull the bottom strap over your head and position it around neck below ears.

**5** Using two hands, mold the nosepiece to the shape of your nose by pushing inward while moving fingertips down both sides of the nosepiece. Pinching the nosepiece using one hand may result in less effective respirator performance.

**6** FACE FIT CHECK
The respirator seal should be checked before each use. To check fit, place both hands completely over the respirator and exhale. If air leaks around your nose, adjust the nosepiece as described in step 5. If air leaks at respirator edges, adjust the straps back along the sides of your head. Recheck.

**NOTE:** If you cannot achieve proper fit, do not enter the isolation or treatment area. See your supervisor.

### Removal instructions:

**1** Cup the respirator in your hand to maintain position on face. Pull bottom strap over head.

**2** Still holding respirator in position, pull top strap over head.

**3** Remove respirator from face and discard or store according to your facility s policy.

**FIGURE 5-13** Fit-test the respirator each time you wear it. *(Courtesy of 3M Health Care, St. Paul, MN)*

## Eye Protection

Eye protection may be in the form of goggles, glasses with solid side shields, or full face shields. The employee should select the device appropriate to the situation. Many employers require employees to wear eye protection as a precaution when caring for every patient. For this reason, some health care providers have side shields fitted to normal prescription glasses. Although this may

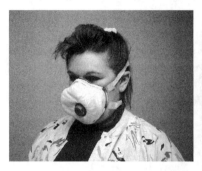
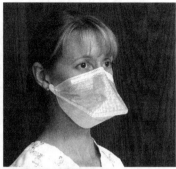
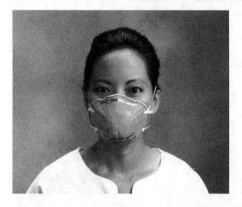

**FIGURE 5-14** Masks should be selected to provide optimal protection for the situation.

meet the requirements set forth by the employer, one should consider the additional protection that safety glasses or goggles may afford in a splash situation.

## Gowns and Protective Apparel

Gowns or additional appropriate cover should be worn in conjunction with other PPE when splash is anticipated. A uniform should not be considered PPE. Appropriate cover must be used to protect the uniform.

Many facilities use paper or plastic gowns for this purpose. Because of the nature of the environment, these gowns may not be appropriate for use in the prehospital or industrial setting. Some prehospital care providers use fluid-resistant paper coveralls or jackets as a more durable option to a gown. Employers should select and purchase protective equipment with the work environment in mind.

# NEWSMAKER
## SARS Outbreak

<u>GENEVA, SWITZERLAND</u>                              MARCH 12, 2003

The World Health Organization (WHO) today announced a global outbreak of an "atypical pneumonia," being referred to as severe acute respiratory syndrome (SARS). The virus, it seems, has been spread internationally along travel routes and has caused well-documented nosocomial outbreaks in Singapore, Hong Kong, Vietnam, China, and Canada.

The Canadian outbreak, which took place in the Greater Toronto area, resulted in 438 cases, including many health care workers. Although droplet and airborne precautions were reportedly taken in affected hospitals, three health care workers died.

In Hong Kong, 40 health care workers in a 529-bed community hospital became infected with SARS over a 6-week period. It was determined that most workers were infected from direct contact with patients with SARS, many of whom were in general wards. Although many workers wore masks when caring for these patients, infection was not suspected at the time.

The causative agent of this outbreak was later found to be a new coronavirus.

1. How might have this outbreak been prevented?

2. As a health care worker, how would you prevent such an exposure?

3. Explain how SARS was spread along "international travel routes."

4. What is a nosocomial infection, and how may one be prevented?

## UNDER THE MICROSCOPE

✿ What precautions should you take when traveling to a country where SARS cases have been reported?
✿ Where did the SARS virus come from?

✿   ✿   ✿

### Uniforms

If a uniform becomes soiled with blood or body fluids, the employer is responsible for its proper cleaning or replacement (at the employer's option). Because of the possibility of cross-contamination of other clothing, the employee should not launder a contaminated uniform at home. Proper laundering requires the use of a front-loading industrial washing machine connected to an approved drainage system.

Commercial laundry facilities may also be used, since they typically use a combination of high water temperatures (>160°F) and chlorine bleach (50–150 parts per million) to ensure the removal of harmful microorganisms. Soiled uniforms should be handled as little as possible and placed in a biohazard bag for transportation to the laundry facility.

If a pull-over shirt is contaminated, it may have to be cut off to avoid unnecessary contact when pulling it over the head. If this is the case, the shirt should be cut off and placed in a biohazard bag for proper disposal. The employee should shower as soon as is practical afterward.

## MEDICAL SUPPLIES AND EQUIPMENT

Medical supplies and equipment should be cleaned, disinfected, and/or sterilized after use. **Cleaning** medical equipment involves removing debris and reducing the number of microorganisms present. Completely immersing the object in liquid or applying a chemical disinfectant to a surface, usually by spraying, accomplishes **disinfection**. Disinfection removes most pathogens, but not their **spores**, which allow for reproduction. **Sterilization** is a process of making an object free from all live microorganisms, usually by gas or steam.

Steps necessary in cleaning medical equipment and instruments include:

1. Apply appropriate personal protective equipment.
2. Ensure that the cleaning agent selected is appropriate and prepared according to manufacturer's recommendations.
3. If applicable, disassemble the instrument to expose all surfaces.
4. Following manufacturer's recommendations, thoroughly clean the instrument.
5. Rinse thoroughly with water.
6. Dry the item and each of its parts.

To disinfect after cleaning, follow these steps:

1. Apply appropriate personal protective equipment.
2. Ensure that the disinfecting agent selected is appropriate and prepared according to manufacturer's recommendations. Verify the concentration of the solution.
3. If applicable, disassemble the instrument to expose all surfaces.
4. If practical, immerse the item in the solution. If not, apply according to manufacturer's recommendations, being careful that the solution contacts all parts of the item. Soak for the recommended time.
5. Rinse at least three times with water.
6. Dry the items thoroughly and reassemble. Compressed air may be used to speed and ensure completion of the drying process.

In 1968, Dr. Earl Spaulding developed the **Spaulding Classification System,** intended to determine appropriate methods for preparing supplies and instruments for patient use based on the item's intended use:

- **Critical**—These are items that penetrate tissue; they must be sterilized.
- **Semicritical**—These are items that contact, but do not penetrate, mucous membranes or nonintact skin. They require a minimum of high-level disinfection.
- **Noncritical**—These are items that contact intact skin, requiring only cleaning and intermediate-level disinfection.

Many medical supplies are disposable and intended for single patient use. These items should be disposed of in an appropriate container after use.

## INTERESTING FACTS

- The cost of follow-up for a high-risk exposure is almost $3000 per needlestick injury, even when no infection occurs.
- One case of serious infection caused by bloodborne pathogens can cost as much as $1 million, according to the American Hospital Association.
- Hepatitis B infections in health care workers have decreased from 17,000 per year before hepatitis B vaccine to 400 per year after OSHA required that employers offer the vaccine.
- 80% of those infected with hepatitis C are asymptomatic.
- Hepatitis C virus is the leading reason for liver transplant.
- There has been only been one case in the United States of a patient being infected with the human immunodeficiency virus (HIV) by a health care provider.

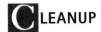

# CLEANUP

When spilled, blood and/or other body fluid should be cleaned up as soon as possible. If broken glass or other sharp objects are involved, care must be taken to ensure that the health care provider does not get cut.

Once appropriate personal protective equipment is donned, care should be taken to contain the spill. One way to achieve this is to cover the spill with paper towels. Once contained, the spill may be absorbed with additional paper towels and placed in a biohazard bag for disposal. A mixture of common household bleach (5.25% sodium hypochlorite diluted with water to between 1:10 and 1:100 should be used to further disinfect the affected area.

## ALERT

Since hepatitis B can remain active for several days in dried blood, care must be taken even when cleaning up dried blood.

# PERSONAL HEALTH

**Personal health** is a three-part system that is a joint responsibility of both the employer and employee. This system includes physical examinations, vaccinations, and return-to-work authorizations.

## Physical Exams

Once hired, the employer should arrange for a **pre-entry physical exam** at no cost to the employee. This exam should screen for infectious disease, answer medical questions that would screen for preexisting illnesses, and help to determine if the employee meets the **essential functions** of the position for which he/she has applied.

Diagnostic tests for hepatitis B, tuberculosis, and other diseases may be performed according to local needs. Many employers offer a battery of laboratory tests to assist the employee in identifying potential health problems. In recent years, many employers have offered memberships to health clubs, and some have placed fitness equipment in-house to encourage the personal fitness of their employees.

**ALERT**

The system of personal health may be effective only when it is comprehensive. Each of the three parts is required to provide maximum protection to the health care provider.

## Vaccinations

Immunizations against common infectious disease should be taken by all employees at risk of occupational exposure to blood and body fluid. The employee should ascertain that immunizations against tetanus, measles, mumps, and rubella are up to date. Boosters should be taken for any immunizations that are not current. A listing of vaccinations recommended for health care providers is shown in Figure 5-15.

| Immunization is Strongly Recommended | Immunization May Be Indicated |
|---|---|
| Hepatitis B | Hepatitis A |
| Influenza | Meningococcal Disease |
| Measles, Mumps, and Rubella | Pertussis |
| Varicella | Typhoid |
| | Smallpox (Vaccinia) |

**FIGURE 5-15** Recommended immunizations for health care providers. (*Source:* Centers for Disease Control and Prevention.)

## Hepatitis B Vaccine

The Occupational Safety and Health Administration (OSHA) requires that employers offer the hepatitis B virus (HBV) vaccine free of charge to Category I employees, who may be at risk of occupational exposure to blood and potentially infectious material. If the employee refuses the vaccine he/she must sign a standard declination form but may opt to take the vaccination at a later date, at the employer's expense.

The vaccination should be offered at a time and place convenient to the employee. Many employers allow employees to receive the vaccine while on duty. If the employee receives the vaccine while off duty, the employer may compensate the employee for time and/or travel expenses, if applicable. The intent of OSHA is that the employer must not make receiving the vaccine inconvenient for the employee.

The HBV vaccine is typically given in a series of 3 intramuscular injections. The first injection is followed by the second in 1 month. The third, and final, dose is given 6 months after the initial dose. Research has shown that immunity is best in young children (100% in ages 0–1) but is very good (average of 98%) in adults. Figure 5-16 graphically represents the chance for immunity after receiving the Recombivax HB hepatitis B vaccine.

Side effects of synthetic vaccines are minimal. The most common side effect is soreness at the injection site. Some people report flu-like symptoms that mimic the symptoms of the disease itself. Persons who are pregnant, nursing an infant, or sensitive to yeast or its components should not receive the vaccine.

## Return-to-Work Authorization

An employee should be released by a physician to return to work after exposure to a communicable disease or after

| Infants | 0–12 months | 100% |
| Children | 1–10 years | 99% |
| Adolescents | 11–20 years | 99% |
| Young Adults | 20–29 years | 98% |
| Adults | 20–39 years | 94% |
| Adults | over 40 years | 89% |

**FIGURE 5-16** Immunity to hepatitis B after administration of Recombivax HB. (*Source*: Merck Vaccine Division. Recombivax HB is a registered trademark of Merck.)

having been absent due to illness or injury. In some cases, the physician's discretion will allow the employee to return to work even while laboratory tests are pending. In a case in which an employee is exposed to the blood or body fluid of a known HIV or HBV carrier, the employee may be reassigned to duty that does not include direct patient contact while awaiting the results of follow-up testing.

 **ALERT**

Some states have an infected health care worker act, which requires health care providers to report if they become infected with a reportable disease.

Postexposure follow-up allows the employee to return to normal duty as soon as practical without exposing patients to undue risk. The employer must not terminate or demote an employee based on recommendations of a physician to limit the employee's activity to that which does not involve direct patient care. Even when employees return to work after having a cold or flu, the employer should have standard procedures for determining their ability to resume normal work duties.

## CONCLUSION

Personal health is an important responsibility shared by the employer and the employee. Both must know their roles and each must work with the other to ensure safety for employees and patients, and to limit liability for the employer.

## QUESTIONS FOR DISCUSSION

1. List at least four examples of common engineering controls.
2. List at least four examples of safe work practices.
3. Who is responsible for ensuring that safe work practices are enforced?
4. Describe the differences in standard precautions and transmission-based precautions.
5. List and describe the three major types of transmission-based precautions.
6. Explain why body substance isolation (BSI) is generally the preferred method of isolation used by pre-hospital and out-of-hospital providers.
7. Who is responsible for laundering or disposing of uniforms contaminated with blood or other potentially infectious materials?
8. List and describe the three components of the personal health system.
9. List the contraindications of the hepatitis B vaccine.
10. Explain the procedure for cleaning up spilled blood.
11. Describe the three categories set forth by the Spaulding Classification System.
12. Differentiate between cleaning, disinfecting, and sterilizing.

## WORTH THINKING ABOUT

- What engineering controls at your agency/institution could be improved?
- Do you sometimes take shortcuts with safe work practices? What are the possible consequences of these shortcuts?
- What do you consider to be the most important safe work practice? Why?

## WEB RESOURCES

**Centers for Disease Control and Prevention**—For timely information on protection from communicable disease, visit the CDC website. http://www.cdc.gov.

**Occupational Safety and Health Administration**—The OSHA site provides a great deal of information on protecting oneself from exposure to infectious disease. http://www.osha.gov.

**American Nursing Association**—This website provides much information on protection from exposure to infectious disease. Download the Needlestick Prevention Guide. http://www.nursingworld.org.

**Association for Professionals in Infection Control and Epidemiology**—The APIC site provides a wealth of information. http://www.apic.org.

## BIBLIOGRAPHY

Acello, B. (1998). *Patient care: Basic skills for the health care provider.* Clifton Park, NY: Thomson Delmar Learning.

American Nurses Association. (2002). *Needlestick prevention guide.* Washington, DC: Author.

Association for Professionals in Infection Control and Epidemiology. http://www.apic.org.

Bolyard, E. A., et al. (1998). Guideline for infection control in health care personnel. *American Journal of Infection Control, 26.*

Centers for Disease Control and Prevention. (2002, October 25). Guideline for hand hygiene in health-care settings. *Morbidity and Mortality Weekly Report, 51.*

Centers for Disease Control and Prevention (2002). *Hand hygiene guidelines fact sheet.* http://www.cdc.gov.

Centers for Disease Control and Prevention. (1998, May 15). Public health service guidelines for the management of health-care worker exposures to HIV and recommendations for postexposure prophylaxis. *Morbidity and Mortality Weekly Report, 47.*

Ho, A. S., et al. (October 7, 2003). An outbreak of severe acute respiratory syndrome among hospital workers in a community hospital in Hong Kong. *Annals of Internal Medicine, 139* (7).

National Fire Academy. (1992). *Infection control for emergency response personnel: The supervisor's role.* Emmitsburg, MD: Author.

National Institute for Occupational Safety and Health. (2004) *NIOSH-approved disposable particulate respirators.* Atlanta: Author.

National Institute for Occupational Safety and Health. (1999). *Preventing needlestick injuries in health care settings.* Atlanta: Author.

National Institute for Occupational Safety and Health. (1998). *Selecting, evaluating, and using sharps disposal containers.* Atlanta: Author.

Offit, P. A., & Bell, L. M. (1999). *Vaccines: What every parent should know.* New York: IDG Books.

Reynolds S. A., Levy F., Walker E.S. Hand sanitizer alert. Emerg Infect Dis 2006 March. Accessed May 1, 2006, from http://www.cdc.gov/ncidod/EID/vol12no03/05-0955.htm.

Romig, L. A., Hudak, D., & Barnard, J. (March, 2005). Scrub or toss? Making the case for disposable laryngoscope blades. *Emergency Medical Services, 34* (3).

The Change Foundation. (2005). *Protecting the faces of health care workers.* Toronto, ON, Canada: Author.

Tokarski, C. (2005). *New CDC recommendations seek to lower nosocomial infections.* http://www.medscape.com.

U.S. Air Force. Web site of the 74th Medical Group, Wright-Patterson Air Force Base.

U.S. Fire Administration. (1992). *Guide to developing and managing an emergency service infection control program.* Washington, DC: Author.

West, K. (2000, Spring). Personal safety solutions. *Emergency Products News,* 8–11.

## CHAPTER 6

# Protection from Infectious Agents Used as Weapons

## LEARNING OBJECTIVES

After completing this chapter, the reader should be able to:

- describe how biological agents have historically been used in warfare and terrorism.
- differentiate between biological terrorism and biological warfare.
- describe the advantages and disadvantages of using biological agents as weapons.
- differentiate between Category A, B, and C agents.
- list six Category A agents.
- list and describe the four components required to make an agent a respirable aerosol.
- explain how to kill most foodborne pathogens.
- explain how to kill most waterborne pathogens.
- describe the health care provider's greatest priority in a bioterrorism incident.

## KEY TERMS

- biological terrorism
- bioterrorism
- biological warfare
- category A agent
- category B agent
- category C agent

- delivery system
- Department of Homeland Security (DHS)
- dissemination device
- foodborne
- microclimate
- public health system
- respirable aerosol
- waterborne

## FEATURED CASE STUDY

| | |
|---|---|
| Date: | September 9, 1984 |
| Patient: | Dan Ericksen |
| Public Health Nurse: | Carla Chamberlain |

Mr. Ericksen, an elected official and leader in his community, presented to his local hospital emergency department reporting stomach cramps, dizziness, chills, fever, vomiting, and diarrhea. He reported that he had eaten from a salad bar at a local pizza restaurant earlier that day. The owners of the restaurant, who had dined with him, were also sick. By the end of the week, dozens of the restaurant's customers and 13 of the restaurant's 28 employees were sick.

1. What do you suspect has happened in this case?
2. Do you suspect terrorism?

Postscript: This outbreak in The Dalles, Oregon, occurred in two waves. The first was September 9 through 18; the second was September 19 through October 10. Most of the cases were associated with 10 restaurants, including the one owned by Dave and Sandy Lutgens, who dined with Dan Ericksen and his family after church on Sunday, September 9. By the time the outbreak was over, 751 people had become ill with *Salmonella* gastroenteritis.

Local, state, and national public health officials investigated all the usual suspects—water supply, food distributor, inadequate refrigeration—but the cause was not found until more than a year later. The cause was determined to be an act of terror perpetrated by a cult called the Rajneeshees. The causative agent, *Salmonella typhimurium*, had been purchased legally from a germ bank that provides pathogens to hospitals and labs for research and diagnostic tests.

## UNDER THE MICROSCOPE

❂ Why do you think terrorists specifically attacked salad bars?

❂ How can you protect yourself from foodborne illnesses when eating in restaurants?

❂ Research more about this incident to discover how the *Salmonella typhimurium* was purchased. What other pathogens had the cult purchased? What would have been the effect of outbreaks of the other agents purchased?

❂  ❂  ❂

# INTRODUCTION

September 11, 2001, changed the world forever. According to experts, a new kind of warfare was born. In November of that same year terrorists experienced some success using anthrax as an instrument of terror. Letters containing anthrax spores were delivered via mail to Capitol Hill offices and to major New York media outlets.

However, using biological agents as weapons is not a new concept. Likewise, the need to protect oneself against these agents has been around for centuries. This chapter will not only highlight the history of biological weapons, but will also describe current threats and how to protect oneself against these threats.

# HISTORY OF BIOLOGICAL AGENTS USED AS WEAPONS

The use of biological agents as weapons may be traced back more than 2000 years, when Scythian archers dipped the heads of their arrows in rotting corpses and manure in an effort to inflict infection on their enemies. The Tatars, in the 14th century, hurled corpses of those who died from plague over the walls of enemy cities in an effort to spread the disease among the enemy.

The British used smallpox during the French and Indian War when they gave unfriendly tribes blankets laced with the disease. During World War I the Germans spread glanders, an equine disease, to enemy calvary forces. In World War II, the Japanese used biological weapons by dropping fleas infected with plague on Chinese cities, killing hundreds.

In the early 20th century, several countries, including the United States, Canada, Germany, Japan, France, and the USSR, either developed or investigated biological weapons programs. Advantages of biological weapons include:

- Their ability to multiply. Those who become infected could spread the agent further.
- Inexpensive compared to traditional weapons and other weapons of mass destruction.
- They are silent killers and can attack with little or no warning.
- They leave property intact.

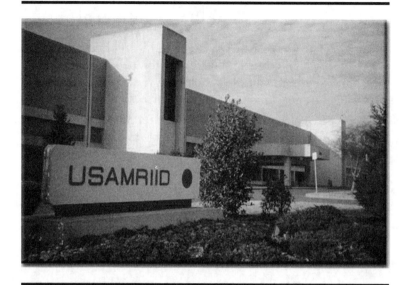

Established in 1969, the U.S. Army Medical Research Institute of Infectious Diseases (USAMRIID) in Fort Detrick, Maryland, has been a focal point of U.S. biological weapons research. (Courtesy: USAMRIID)

A disadvantage of the use of biological agents in warfare, these countries found, is that they are difficult, if not impossible, to control. Once dispersed, a subtle change in wind or weather can turn the agent on those who distributed it or render the agent useless.

 INTERESTING FACTS

- The National Defense University has compiled a study of more than 100 confirmed incidents of illicit use of biological agents during the 1900s.
- The likelihood of someone in the U.S. being infected with plague is 1:287,974,000.

## INTERESTING FACTS (continued)

- The Centers for Disease Control and Prevention (CDC) estimates that 76 million people suffer from foodborne illnesses each year, resulting in 325,000 hospitalizations and more than 5000 deaths.
- In 1979, an explosion at a Soviet bioweapons facility released enough anthrax to kill as many as one thousand people in the city of Sverdlovsk. The secrecy of the Cold War kept details from leaking.
- In the 1980s the U.S. gave Iraq bubonic plague, smallpox, and aerosolized anthrax.
- The U.S. biological weapons program began in 1942.
- Chemical weapons have been around for a long time also. During the Civil War, Dr. Luke Blackburn, who later became governor of Kentucky, sold Union troops clothing contaminated with smallpox and yellow fever. The Union army planned, but never implemented, an attack on the Confederacy using sulfuric and hydrochloric acids.

# CURRENT PERSPECTIVE AND RESOURCES

Since the coordinated September 11, 2001, terrorist attacks on the United States and the anthrax attacks just 2 months later, the United States has focused a great deal of resources to fight terrorism both at home and abroad. The U.S. **Department of Homeland Security (DHS)** was established to coordinate efforts, including training the nation's emergency responders and health care providers to respond to terror attacks. In addition, other agencies, including the CDC, provide a wealth of information and resources on bioterrorism and biological agents.

# NEWSMAKER
## Anthrax Attack!

WASHINGTON, DC                                    OCTOBER 17, 2001

**Senator Daschle's Office and Staffers Test Positive For Anthrax**

After a letter sent to Senator Tom Daschle (D-South Dakota) was found to contain anthrax earlier this week, experts tested Daschle's office and staff today for the presence of anthrax. Thirty-one Capitol workers, including 23 Daschle staffers, five Capitol police officers, and three Russ Feingold staffers tested positive for the presence of anthrax. Feingold's office is located behind Daschle's in the Hart Senate Building. The anthrax found was described as "weapons grade" by the FBI.

Anthrax spores were also found in a Senate mailroom, located in an office building near the Capitol. A photo editor with the tabloid, *The Sun*, recently died in Florida from inhalation anthrax.

Postscript: Five people infected with inhalation anthrax died over the next few weeks and anthrax infections developed in 22. A total of seven letters have been identified as part of the attack, including those sent to Senator Daschle, Senator Patrick Leahy, ABC News, CBS News, NBC News, *The Sun*, and the *New York Post*. No arrests have been made.

1. What precautions should be taken when treating a patient infected with anthrax?

2. One of those who died from anthrax was 94-year-old Ottilie Lundgren, of Oxford, Connecticut. No anthrax was detected in her home. What is the most likely source of her infection? Did her age make her more or less susceptible to anthrax infection?

## UNDER THE MICROSCOPE

❂ Search the Internet to learn more about this terrorist attack. Who died from anthrax? How did they likely become exposed? Were health care providers involved? How could exposure have been prevented?

❂ What post offices were involved? When did they reopen? What took so long?

❂   ❂   ❂

## PROBABLE AGENTS

**Bioterrorism** is the use of viruses, bacteria, or other germs for terrorist purposes. The CDC places biological agents in three categories (A, B, and C) based on their ability to cause harm.

### Category A

**Category A agents** include organisms that risk national security because they can be easily transmitted from person to person, may result in high mortality rates or have major public health impact, may cause public panic, and require special action for public health preparedness. Category A agents include anthrax, botulism, plague, smallpox, tularemia, and viral hemorrhagic fevers.

## Category B

**Category B agents** are second-priority agents that are moderately easy to disseminate, result in moderate morbidity and low mortality rates, and require special enhancements to the CDC's capacity. Agents in this category include brucellosis, food and water safety threats, glanders, psittacosis, and ricin.

## Category C

**Category C agents** are third-priority agents that include emerging pathogens that may be engineered for future mass dissemination based on availability, ease of production, and potential for major health impact and high morbidity and mortality rates. Examples of such pathogens include Nipah virus and hantavirus.

Specific information on many of these agents is included in Appendix A.

# PROBABLE DELIVERY DEVICES

While most military experts agree that biological weapons are not well suited to warfare, they are increasingly being seen as a threat in the hands of terrorists. **Biological warfare** involves the intentional use of bacteria, viruses, or toxins to cause death or disease in humans, plants, or animals. It is usually state-sponsored and delivered in large quantities with great precision by bombs, missiles, or spray systems in an effort to win a war.

**Biological terrorism** is the intentional or threatened used of biological agents to make a statement or to undermine authority. It usually involves a small quantity of agent that can be released at any time, in any location, and against any target.

Devices used to deliver biological weapons vary, depending on the agent. Mass distribution of many biological agents requires that they be presented as a **respirable aerosol**, a gaseous suspension of fine solid or liquid particles that is capable of being inhaled. Aerosol delivery depends on four components:

1. The agent—The agent must be processed so that it may be aerosolized.
2. The delivery system—The **delivery system** is the vehicle, like a plane, truck, or boat, in which the dissemination device is carried.
3. The dissemination device—The **dissemination device** may be in a variety of forms, ranging from a simple low-volume delivery device (like an aerosol can) to a large industrial or agricultural device or even an existing air handling system of a building.
4. The weather or microclimate—The weather is a very important factor in the dissemination of biological agents. Lack of cloud cover, ultraviolet (UV) rays, and rain can adversely affect the efficacy of a biological agent. A **microclimate** refers to the conditions within an area such as a building.

Other methods for disseminating biological agents include contaminating food, water, and livestock. Most of the agents transmitted this way are other than Category A agents. Water treatment is effective against most **waterborne** agents and thorough cooking is effective against most **foodborne** agents.

## PREVENTION AND SURVEILLANCE

Existing **public health systems** are essential in the early detection, recognition, and identification of a biological attack. State and regional laboratories have strengthened their capacity to detect biological agents and to communicate with the CDC. As part of that effort, the CDC has established the Health Alert Network, intended to strengthen the core public health infrastructure for information access, communications, and distance learning at the state and community levels. This network provides vital public health information and the infrastructure to support dissemination of that information to local communities nationwide.

To prepare for outbreaks caused by the release of biological agents, the CDC and pharmaceutical companies have established regional stockpiles of necessary medications. Intelligence and enforcement efforts have been strengthened. The key in containing biological threats is rapid detection and dissemination of information.

## HEALTH CARE PROVIDER SAFETY

Since an ill health care provider can help no one, the first priority for the health care provider in a biological terrorism situation is personal safety. When responding to incidents involving biological agents, health care providers must have the training and personal protective equipment to protect them from contamination.

During routine patient care, standard precautions should be used for all involved patients. Airborne precautions should be taken when appropriate. For agent-specific precautions, see the disease listing in Appendix A.

## CONCLUSION

The odds are not great that a health care provider will be called on to care for a victim of biological terrorism or warfare, but it is important to understand how to protect oneself from exposure to biological agents. The U.S. government has done much to reduce the risk of biological terrorism and to improve detection and response to bioterrorism incidents.

## QUESTIONS FOR DISCUSSION

1. Describe at least three cases in which biological weapons were used in warfare.
2. Compare and contrast bioterrorism and biological warfare in terms of delivery systems, agents, and motive.
3. Why have biological weapons not been used widely in warfare?
4. What are two advantages to biological warfare?
5. Differentiate between Category A, B, and C agents; name at least two examples of each.
6. List the six Category A agents.
7. Describe how to make an agent a respirable aerosol.
8. Faced with a bioterrorism incident, what is your greatest priority?
9. How can you best protect yourself against foodborne pathogens?
10. How can you best protect yourself against waterborne pathogens?

## WORTH THINKING ABOUT

- What buildings in your area are likely terrorist targets? Why?
- Why do terrorists do what they do? Can they be stopped?

## WEB RESOURCES

**University of Alabama in Birmingham Bioterrorism and Emerging Infections Education**—This site provides a great deal of information on bioterrorism agents and emerging infectious diseases. http://www.bioterrorism.uab.edu.

**Centers for Disease Control and Prevention**—This site provides a wealth of information on biological agents. http://www.cdc.gov. Click on "Emergency Preparedness and Response" then on "Bioterrorism Agents."

## BIBLIOGRAPHY

Centers for Disease Control and Prevention web site. (2005).
http://www.cdc.gov.

DeNoon, D. (2004). *Biological and chemical terror history.*
http://www.webmd.com.

Federal Bureau of Investigation. (2001). *The search for anthrax.*
http://www.fbi.gov.

Franz, D. R. (2005). *Bioterrorism: the public health threat* (online course).
University of Alabama in Birmingham Bioterrorism and Emerging
Infections Education. http://www.bioterrorism.uab.edu.

Miller, J., Engelberg, J., & Broad, W. (2002). *Germs: Biological weapons and
America's secret war.* New York: Touchstone.

Sunshine Project. (2005). Some facts about the U.S. biodefense program and
public health. http://www.sunshine-project.org.

Torok, T. J., et al. (1997, August 6). A large community outbreak of
salmonellosis caused by intentional contamination of restaurant salad
bars. *Journal of the American Medical Association, 278* (5).

Wikipedia. 2001 anthrax attacks. http://en.wikipedia.org/wiki/
2001_anthrax_attacks.

## CHAPTER 7

# Exposure Determination

## LEARNING OBJECTIVES

After completing this chapter, the reader should be able to:

- recognize a potential exposure to communicable disease.
- list six components normally required for an exposure to take place.
- discuss two questions health care providers may ask themselves to determine the likelihood of exposure to communicable disease.

## KEY TERMS

- exposure
- method of travel
- mode of transmission
- portal of entry

## FEATURED CASE STUDY

Date:          June 21, 2005
Patient:       Calvin Genheim
Nurse:         Chloe Nived

While working the overnight shift, registered nurse Chloe Nived noticed that Mr. Genheim's intravenous (IV) line had infiltrated and needed to be discontinued and restarted. She applied gloves before removing the existing line, disposed of the IV catheter in a sharps container, and held direct pressure on the site.

As she began making her venipuncture to restart the IV, the patient became startled and jerked his arm, displacing the needle and directing it toward Chloe's left wrist, where it punctured the skin.

1. How will Chloe determine if she was potentially exposed to a communicable disease?
2. In addition to needlesticks, list some other potential portals of entry.

# INTRODUCTION

Potential exposure to communicable disease can be a trying experience. This is why it is important for health care providers to understand what constitutes an exposure and what to do when a potential exposure occurs.

This chapter is not intended as a complete guide to exposure. It should, however, be helpful in determining if an exposure has occurred.

# CHAIN OF INFECTION

The chain of infection (Figure 7-1) illustrates six components necessary for communicable disease to be spread. A brief discussion of each follows.

## Causative Agent

The causative agent of a disease is the virus, bacteria, fungus, rickettsia, or protozoan that causes the disease. For example, the causative agent of acquired immuno-deficiency syndrome (AIDS) is the human immuno-deficiency virus (HIV) and the causative agent of mononucleosis is the Epstein–Barr virus.

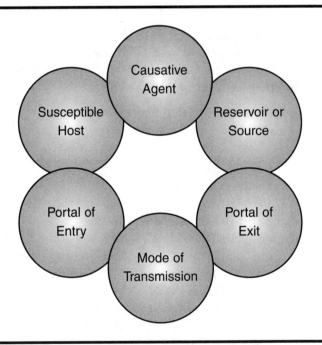

**FIGURE 7-1** Chain of infection.

## Reservoir or Source

Each causative agent must have a place for the source to reside and grow, referred to as a *source* or *reservoir*. This is the person or object that carries the disease. In the case of rabies, the reservoir may be an infected dog. In tetanus, the source may be a rusty nail. It is important that health care providers isolate themselves from the source or potential reservoirs of infectious disease.

## Portal of Exit

For the pathogen to transfer from the carrier to a susceptible host there must be a portal of exit. In other words, there must be some way for the pathogen to leave the body of the carrier. This may be through a sneeze or cough, or through blood or other potentially infectious materials. A review of transmission methods is in Chapter 3.

## Mode of Transmission

As discussed in Chapter 3, transmission may be accomplished through a variety of methods. The goal of the health care provider should be to prevent transmission through the use of appropriate personal protective equipment.

## Portal of Entry

For exposure to take place, the causative agent must find its way into the body of the exposed person. The way the pathogen enters the body is referred to as the portal of entry. Without a portal of entry, there is no exposure.

## Susceptible Host

The final requirement for exposure is a susceptible host. This means that the potentially exposed person must be susceptible to the disease. Health care providers may reduce their chance of susceptibility by maintaining a general state of health and being immunized against infectious diseases.

# NEWSMAKER
## City Supports Firefighters

PHILADELPHIA, PA                                    JANUARY 27, 2000

**City Will Support Firefighters/
Paramedics**

Mayor John F. Street announced earlier this week that the city would commit enough money to treat up to 200 firefighters and paramedics who have contracted the hepatitis C virus. Up to $3 million dollars will be set aside this year for this purpose.

The union reports that 130 firefighter/paramedics, or 6% of the department's members, have contracted hepatitis C, a bloodborne virus affecting the liver. It is expected that these firefighters were exposed to the disease while on duty, since many of those infected have been working with the department for decades.

Unfortunately, the time of exposure cannot be pinpointed, since infection control in the prehospital setting was not an issue until the mid- to late 1980s. And since hepatitis C can remain dormant for many years, those who became infected did not know they were sick. Signs and symptoms of hepatitis C mimic those of the flu, so even if symptoms were present, those infected may have just thought they had the flu.

Follow-up: Firefighters and paramedics in other cities became infected with the virus. Just 2 months after this report 10 to 15 San Francisco firefighters and at least 10 more Philadelphia fire department members had been diagnosed with the virus. Three had died.

1. Though infectious disease exposure did not garner much attention until the mid-1980s, do you expect that standard operating procedures were in place prior to then that, if followed, would have documented exposure incidents?

2. How would these exposures be documented today?

3. Since the signs and symptoms of hepatitis C mimic those of the flu, do you expect that those infected may have experienced some symptoms over the years?

## UNDER THE MICROSCOPE

❂ Follow up on this story to learn how many firefighters are now infected and how many have died. Try to discover if other cities have experienced similar infection rates among firefighters.

❂ Look up the hepatitis C infection rate for the general public and health care workers and compare that to the infection rate for Philadelphia Fire Department.

❂   ❂   ❂

# EXPOSURE IN A NUTSHELL

Some of the components in the chain of infection may be difficult to measure. For that reason, a basic discussion of exposure follows. Although exposure is not as simple as the following definition, this section may be helpful in determining whether a health care provider has been exposed to a communicable disease.

In simple terms, **exposure** to communicable disease requires two components. The first component is a **method of travel** or mode of transmission. A **mode of transmission** is the means through which the pathogen enters the body. In a needlestick incident, the needle is the method of travel. The infected material travels from the host patient to the employee by way of the needle. Common methods of travel are through needles and through direct contact with blood and/or body fluid.

The second component required in an exposure is the **portal of entry.** This is the path through which the infected material gains entry into the body. In a needlestick incident, the place where the needle punctures the skin is the portal of entry for the disease. Common portals of entry

| Situation | Portal of Entry | Method of Travel | Exposure? |
|---|---|---|---|
| Your glove tears and you get blood on your fingers. You have no cuts on your hands. | There is no portal of entry. | Yes, through the blood. | No, since there was no portal of entry. |
| Blood is splattered into your eye from a patient. | Yes, through the mucous membranes around the eyes. | Yes, through the blood. | Yes, there was a portal of entry and a mode of transmission. |

FIGURE 7-2 Exposure situations. This figure illustrates how both portal of entry and mode of transmission are important in assessing a possible exposure.

include punctures from needlesticks, nonintact or dry, cracked skin, and absorption through mucous membranes.

These two components should be considered when assessing the possibility of exposure. The absence of either factor is a good indication that no exposure took place. Figure 7-2 illustrates this point.

# AIRBORNE EXPOSURE

Exposure to airborne disease is often difficult to determine. An exposure occurs when droplets from a sneeze or cough are inhaled or deposited in an area of mucous membranes. These areas are highly vascular and may absorb contaminants into the bloodstream.

Exposure is also possible when an employee comes in contact with a patient in confined or close quarters. For this reason, persons who provide care to someone with an active airborne transmissible disease in close quarters, such as in the back of an ambulance, are considered to have been potentially exposed. Because of the proximity of the patient and the health care provider, exposure is assumed even if there is no definable exposure incident.

## INTERESTING FACTS

O As many as 27% of those in the United States infected with HIV/AIDS do not know they are infected.

O There are more than 12 million health care workers in the U.S., 80% of whom are female.

O Occupational injury rates in the health care sector have increased over the past decade. In contrast, occupational injury rates in the two most dangerous sectors, agriculture and construction, have decreased.

O According to Johns Hopkins University Medical School, as many as 87% of surgeons will, during their career, receive an occupational injury that breaks the skin.

## CONCLUSION

When assessing a possible exposure, it is important to note both the portal of entry and the mode of transmission. If an employee believes he/she has been exposed, the incident should be reported to his/her supervisor as soon as practical. The supervisor should be taught and equipped to assist the employee in determining whether an exposure took place, and in providing appropriate emergency care and documentation of the exposure incident. Chapter 8 covers what should be done once an exposure has occurred.

## QUESTIONS FOR DISCUSSION

1. Why is it harder to determine exposure to airborne transmitted diseases than exposure to bloodborne transmitted diseases?

2. What two things are necessary to prove an exposure occurred?

3. Why would someone who rides in an ambulance carrying a patient with an airborne communicable disease be considered to have been exposed? Would someone who rides in a car with that same person be considered exposed? Why or why not?

## WORTH THINKING ABOUT

- Consider what your first emotion might be after an exposure takes place.
- How can you assist a coworker who has been exposed to blood or other potentially infectious material?

## WEB RESOURCES

**Infection Control Today**—This is the website for *Infection Control Today*, one of the leading infection control publications. http://www.infectioncontroltoday.com.

**National Institutes of Health**—The NIH website provides a wealth of information, including model exposure control plans. Search for "exposure control." http://www.nih.gov.

## BIBLIOGRAPHY

Acello, B. (1998). *Patient care: Basic skills for the health care provider*. Clifton Park, NY: Thomson Delmar Learning.

Associated Press. (2000, January 24). Philly to provide for hepatitis C: Mayor offers millions for treatment. *Firehouse.com Third Alarm News*.

Brown, J. K. (2000, March 27). Hep C is deadly: Many emergency workers around country afraid to be tested or treated. *Firehouse.com Third Alarm News*.

Centers for Disease Control and Prevention. (1989, June 23). Guidelines for prevention of transmission of human immunodeficiency virus and hepatis B virus to health-care and public safety workers. *Morbidity and Mortality Weekly Report, 38* (S-6).

Makary, M. A., et al. (2005, May). Scalpel-free surgery could reduce risk of HIV and hepatitis for health care workers in city hospitals. Accessed April 26, 2006, from http://www.hopkinsmedicine.org/Press_releases/2005/05_04_05.html.

U.S. Department of Labor, Occupational Safety and Health Administration. (1991, Dec. 6). *Occupational exposure to bloodborne pathogens.* CFR 1910.1030, Final Rule.

U.S. Department of Labor, Occupational Safety and Health Administration. (1992). *Occupational exposure to bloodborne pathogens: Precautions for emergency responders.* OSHA 3130.

## CHAPTER 8

# Post Exposure

## LEARNING OBJECTIVES

After completing this chapter, the reader should be able to:

- identify where written postexposure protocols are found in his/her place of employment.
- list the steps that should be taken after an exposure.
- understand that confidential medical records must be maintained for exposure incidents.
- understand how to access outside assistance in dealing with postexposure follow-up.
- discuss why exposure may be stressful.
- list at least three ways to reduce stress.

## KEY TERMS

- exposure report form
- first aid
- postexposure testing and follow-up
- prophylaxis
- return-to-work authorization

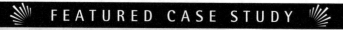

**FEATURED  CASE  STUDY**

Date:              March 21, 2006
Patient:           Hans Genheim
Nursing Assistant: Rudy Santella

Rudy Santella, a certified nursing assistant, was working the night shift at Golden Years Convalescent and Rehabilitation Center when he encountered Mr. Genheim, a resident who had been admitted with traumatic brain injury, actively seizing on the floor beside his bed. Santella pushed the call button to summon the nurse and began to clear the area around Mr. Genheim, hoping to protect him from injury. The nurse arrived with a shot of diazepam, which she gave intramuscularly. Just as the seizing ceased, the patient's arm jerked, knocking the nurse's hand and the syringe toward Rudy's right knee. The needle entered his leg just above his knee.

1. Has Rudy been exposed? Why or why not?
2. What should be Rudy's first action?
3. What documentation is required?
4. How long must the exposure records be kept by the employer?

# INTRODUCTION

Each employer should develop written protocols that guide employees through the exposure-reporting process. These protocols are an integral part of the employer's exposure control plan and must be accessible to each employee who is at risk of occupational exposure. This chapter defines general guidelines for immediate response following an occupational exposure. Employees should become familiar with and follow protocols as published in the employer's exposure control plan.

## FIRST AID

The first priority following an exposure is to take immediate **first aid** measures. This includes bleeding control, wound cleansing and dressing, and/or flushing the eyes as appropriate. Other, more advanced, first aid may be indicated and should be performed by appropriately trained personnel.

Simple wounds should be cleaned with soap and water. Dry, sterile dressings should be applied and held in place with bandages. If the eyes are affected, they may be washed in a commercial eye wash station or with an improvised eye wash. (See Figure 8-1 for instructions.) If neither is available, the eyes should be washed with ordinary tap water for a minimum of 20 minutes.

## REPORTING

All exposures should be reported to the employee's immediate supervisor as soon as practical following an exposure incident. However, first aid measures take priority and should not be delayed in an attempt to notify the employee's supervisor.

An **exposure report form** must be completed for each exposure and filed with the supervisor as directed in the employer's exposure control plan. The supervisor should then route the form to the designated officer who will assist the employee with **postexposure testing and follow-up.** Although medical records related to exposure are not kept in the employee's personnel record, exposure

### Improvised Eye Wash

*Items Needed:*

| | |
|---|---|
| 1 or more | bags of normal saline |
| 1 | nasal cannula |
| 1 | macrodrip (standard) intravenous (IV) tubing |

*TIP:* When flushing the eyes, encourage the patient to keep his/her eyes open and to alternately look in all directions. This will allow all exposed areas of the eyes and the surrounding membranes to be washed.

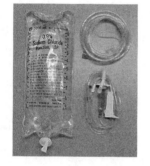

*Directions:*

1. Spike the bag of normal saline just as you would in preparation to start an IV line.

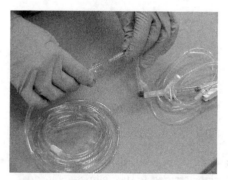

2. Attach the oxygen connector end of the nasal cannula to the distal end of the IV tubing.

3. Place patient in a supine or reclining position and place the prongs of the nasal cannula over the bridge of the nose so one prong is pointed toward each eye. Open the flow control valve on the IV tubing and adjust flow rate to keep a constant flood of saline in the eyes.

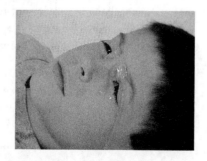

**FIGURE 8-1** Eye wash instructions. This effective eye wash may be constructed with common items.

reports and medical follow-up records must be kept for the length of employment plus 30 years.

# TESTING

The designated officer will coordinate whatever testing and treatment is deemed necessary by the attending physician. The physician may test for the human immunodeficiency virus (HIV), hepatitis B virus (HBV), and hepatitis C virus (HCV) or may prescribe medications as **prophylaxis** for other diseases (Figure 8-2). The Occupational Safety and Health Administration (OSHA) requires that all confidential medical records resulting from an exposure be maintained separately from employment records.

---

**National Clinicians' Post-Exposure Prophylaxis Hotline (PEPline)**
1-888-448-4911
24 hours a day

The PEPline was established to help clinicians counsel and treat health care providers who have occupational exposure to bloodborne diseases. It is staffed by physicians trained to give clinicians information, counseling, and treatment recommendations for health care providers who have received needlestick injuries or other serious occupational exposure to bloodborne pathogens.

The PEPline is a service of the Centers for Disease Control and Prevention and the Health Resources and Services Administration in collaboration with the University of California, San Francisco, and the San Francisco Department of Public Health.

---

**FIGURE 8-2** National Clinicians' Post-Exposure Prophylaxis Hotline (PEPline). (*Source:* Centers for Disease Control and Prevention.)

# OSHA REPORTING REQUIREMENTS

OSHA, through the Needlestick Safety and Prevention Act, requires that employers who are required to maintain a log of occupational injuries and illnesses under 29 CFR 1904 also establish and maintain a sharps injury log to record percutaneous injuries from contaminated sharps. This log must be maintained in a manner that protects the confidentiality of the injured employee and must contain, at a minimum:

- The date of the incident.
- The work area or department where the injury occurred.
- The type and brand of device involved in the incident.
- An explanation of how the incident occurred.

The logs must be maintained for at least 5 years following the end of the calendar years that they cover. Annual review of the log will help employers to identify departments, procedures, and devices involved in injuries.

It is generally accepted that employers who have 10 or more employees at any time during the previous calendar year are required to maintain a log of occupational injuries and illnesses, although some variances may apply. States with their own plans must have standards at least as stringent as the OSHA standards.

### ALERT

Since OSHA requires that some injuries (those involving fatalities or multiple hospitalizations) be reported regardless of the size of the company, the employer may want to consider voluntary compliance with OSHA reporting standards set forth in 29 CFR 1904.

# NEWSMAKER
## Ford Calls for $135 Million

WASHINGTON, DC                                      MARCH 24, 1976

**President Ford Calls for Congress to Appropriate $135 Million for Swine Flu Vaccine**

President Gerald R. Ford today announced that he would ask Congress to appropriate $135 million for the production of "sufficient vaccine to inoculate every man, woman, and child in the United States" against swine flu. With Albert Sabin and Jonas Salk at his side, the president told the nation that he didn't know how serious the threat (of a swine flu pandemic) could be.

The scare started on February 4, when an 18-year-old recruit at Fort Dix, New Jersey, who although he had been reporting aches and pains, fever, and running nose, and had been sent to bed, decided to take a 5-mile hike with his unit. As he marched, his breathing difficulty increased until he collapsed. He died a few hours later in the hospital. The cause of death was listed as influenza complicated by pneumonia.

For the past month others at Fort Dix had reported similar symptoms. Most ignored the symptoms and continued their training. CDC researchers identified the causative agent of the disease as a swine flu virus, very similar to the virus that was thought to have caused a flu pandemic in 1918, which killed millions worldwide. Researchers believed that the 1918 virus, which had infected pigs since 1918, had been spread to humans and was now being spread person to person.

Postscript: About 40 million people received the swine flu vaccine before the program was shelved as unnecessary. No pandemic emerged.

1. Can you think of other disease outbreaks that frightened the public?

2. How may one reduce the risk of exposure to influenza?

3. What should you do if you believe you were exposed to an airborne communicable disease at work?

## UNDER THE MICROSCOPE

❂ Research the 1918 flu pandemic to learn more about this incredible pandemic. An excellent resource is *Flu: The Story of the Great Influenza Pandemic of 1918 and the Search for the Virus That Caused It* by Gina Kolata.

❂ Ask someone you know (who would remember 1976) if they received the swine flu vaccine. Ask them to tell you what they remember about the disease, the inoculation process, and the media coverage.

❂   ❂   ❂

# RETURN TO WORK

The **return-to-work authorization** may authorize an employee to return to normal job duties or it may limit the employee to duties that do not involve direct patient contact. The Americans with Disabilities Act (ADA) specifically names infectious disease as a disability that employers must not discriminate against. It might be unwise to place a person with a known communicable disease in a setting of direct patient care; however, it would be discriminatory to terminate an individual's employment based on a disability. Often, persons who are unable to return to duties involving direct patient care are reassigned in areas where exposure is less likely.

OSHA requires that the employer obtain and provide to the employee a copy of the physician's written opinion within 15 days of completion of the medical evaluation. The content of this report must include a statement that the employee has been informed of the results of the postexposure evaluation and told about medical conditions resulting from the exposure incident that may require further evaluation and treatment. Any other findings must remain confidential and may not be contained in the written report.

# Managing Stress

Even if no disease is contracted, exposure to communicable disease can be highly stressful to an individual and his/her spouse or significant other and/or family. Employers should recognize the needs of employees and their families and provide appropriate counseling to help them cope with the stress of an exposure.

### ALERT

Health care providers should be alert to signs of stress in their coworkers.

The offer of counseling by the employer is sometimes not enough. Health care providers have a responsibility to recognize their stress and the stress of their loved ones. Common signs and symptoms of stress include irritability, fatigue, lack of concentration, insomnia, and depression. See Figure 8-3 for a more comprehensive listing.

| Physical Changes | Emotional Changes |
|---|---|
| Headaches | Lack of concentration |
| Shortness of breath | Irritability |
| Increased pulse rate | Anger |
| Nausea | Mood swings |
| Insomnia | Overreactivity |
| Fatigue | Depression |
| Neck or back pain | Eating disorders |
| Dermatological problems | Anxiety |
| Chronic constipation/diarrhea | Low self-image |
| | Hopeless feelings |

FIGURE 8-3 Physical and emotional signs of stress.

People choose to cope with stress in different ways. Before one may combat stress, however, its presence must first be recognized. Once this is accomplished, the health care provider may use a combination of counseling, education, and physical strategies to help reduce stress levels.

## Counseling

Counseling sessions with a mental health professional may help the health care provider and his or her family cope with the uncertainties of exposure. Participation in peer support groups and/or informal peer counseling may also prove helpful.

## Education

Learning more about the disease process may also help the health care provider cope with exposure. It is also important to educate the family of an exposed health care professional so they will understand the implications of exposure and the process of testing and follow-up. OSHA requires that postexposure counseling include recommendations for prevention of HIV, including refraining from blood or organ donation, abstaining from sexual intercourse, and refraining from breast-feeding infants during the follow-up period.

## Physical Strategies

Counseling and education deal with the psychological aspect of stress management, but it is also important that exposed health care providers use physical strategies that help reduce stress. This includes getting adequate rest, participation in leisure activities, and exercise. Physical exercise may relieve both muscle tension and mental tension, and may cause the release of endorphins, the body's own mood-elevating chemicals.

Good nutrition is also essential to stress reduction and overall good health. For best results, health care providers should eat well-balanced diets, limit their consumption of caffeine, and drink plenty of water each day.

Although many health care providers may find it hard to do so, they should also learn to relax. Many relaxation techniques are available, including breathing exercises, yoga, and meditation. Some people find relaxation in activities like gardening, fishing, golfing, and painting. Whether your idea of relaxation is resting in a hammock or running a marathon, it is important that you take the time to relax and rejuvenate your body, especially during times of extreme physical and/or emotional stress.

## CONCLUSION

Postexposure reporting and medical follow-up is an unpleasant chore at best, but cooperation between the employer and the employee can make the process of testing and waiting more bearable. Health care providers can help themselves and their families by understanding the signs and symptoms of stress and using strategies for stress reduction.

## QUESTIONS FOR DISCUSSION

1. How long must exposure records be kept by the employer?
2. What is the first priority after an exposure?
3. Can an employer fire an employee for contracting a communicable disease while off duty?
4. List at least five signs or symptoms of stress.
5. Discuss several strategies for stress reduction.

## WORTH THINKING ABOUT

- Consider the stress you and your loved ones might experience should you become exposed to a communicable disease.
- What is the most effective relaxation technique for you? What do other members of your family do for stress relief?

## WEB RESOURCES

**Occupational Safety and Health Administration** — This site provides a wealth of resources on a variety of workplace health topics, including exposure to communicable disease. http://www.osha.gov.

**American Nurses Association** — Although this site is designed primarily for the nursing profession, it also contains resources, such as the *ANA's Needlestick Prevention Guide*, that can be used by any health care provider. http://www.nursingworld.org.

**University of California at San Francisco** — UCSF sponsors PEPline, which provides 24/7 access to clinicians who will answer your questions about postexposure prophylaxis. http://www.ucsf.edu. Search "PEPline."

## BIBLIOGRAPHY

Acello, B. (1998). *Patient care: Basic skills for the health care provider*. Clifton Park, NY: Thomson Delmar Learning.

Colbert, B. J. (2000). *Workplace readiness for health occupations*. Clifton Park, NY: Thomson Delmar Learning.

Department of Health and Human Services. Website. http://www.dhhs.gov.

Kolata, G. (2001). *Flu: The story of the great influenza pandemic of 1918 and the search for the virus that caused it*. New York: Touchstone.

National Fire Academy. (1992). *Infection control for emergency response personnel: The supervisor's role*. Emmitsburg, MD: Author.

U.S. Fire Administration. (1992). *Guide to developing and managing an emergency service infection control program*. Washington, DC: Author.

# APPENDIX A

# Diseases of Concern

## INTRODUCTION

This appendix is a quick reference for the health care provider. The information contained within may be considered an overview of the various diseases covered. The reader is encouraged to seek additional resources about a variety of infectious diseases not listed here.

Each disease listed includes information on the **causative agent**, or what bacteria, virus, fungus, protozoa, or rickettsia causes the disease. Next, the body systems typically affected by the disease are shown, followed by a brief description of who, if anyone, is most **susceptible** to this particular disease. Routes of transmission are discussed, as are common signs and symptoms, and patient treatment procedures. Next, protective measures that should be taken by the health care provider are listed, followed by the availability of a vaccine for the disease. Finally, the incubation period for the disease is listed and a section labeled HEALTH CARE PROVIDERS lists information of specific interest to health care providers.

## LIST OF DISEASES

130

The icons shown in Figure A-1 are used to facilitate ease of use.

Health care provider alert

Vaccine available

**FIGURE A-1** These icons will be used throughout this appendix as a quick reference for the reader.

## ACQUIRED IMMUNODEFICIENCY SYNDROME (AIDS)

**Causative Agent**

AIDS is caused by the human immunodeficiency virus (HIV), specifically HIV-1 and HIV-2. HIV-1 is far more pathogenic than HIV-2. Most known cases are HIV-1 Group M.

**Body Systems Affected**

HIV primarily affects the immune system and may also affect the nervous, respiratory, and integumentary systems.

**Susceptibility**

Persons with preexisting sexually transmitted diseases (STDs), those who have unprotected sex with multiple partners, and intravenous drug users who share needles are at increased risk of contracting the HIV virus.

**Routes of Transmission**

HIV may be transmitted through unprotected sexual contact, sharing intravenous needles, and needlesticks.

**Signs and Symptoms**

Signs and symptoms vary but may include fatigue, night sweats, fever, diarrhea, swollen lymph nodes, skin lesions (Figure A-2), and unexplained weight loss. The HIV-infected patient may remain **asymptomatic** for months or years.

**Patient Treatment**

Care is primarily supportive. Treat signs and symptoms.

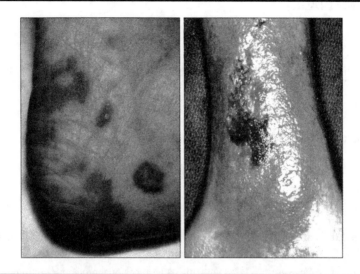

**FIGURE A-2** Kaposi's sarcoma. This cancer of the blood vessels, which causes reddish-purple skin lesions, may be found in patients with HIV.

**Protective Measures**    Standard precautions are indicated. Be especially careful when handling any blood or blood-containing body fluids.

**Immunizations**    There is no vaccine available for HIV or AIDS at this time.

**Incubation Period**    The incubation period for HIV may be up to 10 years.

**Health Care Providers**    Although occupational exposure to HIV is rare, health care providers should isolate themselves from contact with blood or blood-containing body fluids. Since HIV does not survive long outside the human body, the greatest risk for transmission to health care providers is through a needlestick.

## AMEBIASIS

| | |
|---|---|
| **Causative Agent** | Amebiasis is caused by a microscopic parasite called *Entamoeba histolytica*. |
| **Body Systems Affected** | This parasitic disease affects the gastrointestinal system. |
| **Susceptibility** | Susceptibility is general, although those who visit tropical climates are more likely to be exposed. |
| **Routes of Transmission** | Transmission can be person to person through contact with fecal material, by drinking contaminated water, or by eating contaminated food. |
| **Signs and Symptoms** | Most experience few, if any symptoms. Symptoms, if they appear, are typically mild and may include nausea, diarrhea, and abdominal pain. |
| **Patient Treatment** | Treatment is generally supportive. Antibiotics and intravenous fluid therapy may be indicated. |
| **Protective Measures** | As with any patient, personal protective equipment (PPE) should be used, and hand washing should be thorough. |
| **Immunizations** | There is no immunization for amebiasis at this time. |
| **Incubation Period** | Incubation period for amebiasis may be from a few days to a few months. The typical incubation period is 2 to 4 weeks. |
| **Health Care Providers** | Health care providers should use standard precautions and avoid contact with fecal material. |

## ANTHRAX (WOOLSORTERS' DISEASE)

| | |
|---|---|
| **Causative Agent** | Anthrax is a bacterial disease that can infect any warm-blooded animal, including humans. |
| **Body Systems Affected** | Anthrax affects the integumentary, lymphatic, and respiratory systems. |
| **Susceptibility** | Although anthrax may be used as a biological weapon, it is typically considered an occupational disease for those who have exposure to dead animals and animal products. |
| **Routes of Transmission** | Anthrax may be spread by handling contaminated wool or hair or by eating undercooked meat from diseased animals. Anthrax may also live in the soil |

and may be transmitted by inhaling contaminated soil particles.

**Signs and Symptoms**

Signs and symptoms vary with the type of exposure. Exposure to the skin can cause boil-like lesions. Inhalation of anthrax may cause symptoms that resemble a cold and may progress to respiratory distress or failure.

**Patient Treatment**

Care is supportive, with an emphasis on ventilatory support. Penicillin or tetracycline may he helpful.

**Protective Measures**

There are no reported cases of anthrax being spread person to person. However, opportunity for exposure to the health care provider exists when the source of the disease may be present. In that case, respiratory protection is indicated along with standard precautions.

**Immunizations**

There is a vaccine for anthrax, which is recommended for those who work in occupations with potential for exposure.

**Incubation Period**

The incubation period of anthrax is usually less than 7 days.

**Health Care Providers**

Health care providers should be cautious on two fronts. When treating persons with potential occupational exposure to anthrax, health care providers should use barriers to prevent exposure to potentially contaminated materials. Care should also be taken to decontaminate the patient.

In today's world, health care providers should also be aware of the potential for the use of anthrax as a biological weapon. Rapid recognition of the signs and symptoms of anthrax in a multiple-patient situation coupled with the everyday practice of standard precautions could help avert a major incident.

## AVIAN (BIRD) INFLUENZA

**Causative Agent**

Avian flu is caused by the H5N1 virus, an influenza A virus subtype that occurs naturally and is carried in the intestinal system of wild birds. Although this influenza does not normally make wild birds sick, it is highly contagious among birds and can infect, sicken, and kill domesticated birds. It is not common, but it can also be transmitted from birds to humans. The fear is that H5N1 could mutate and have the ability to be spread person-to-person, causing a worldwide pandemic.

**Body Systems Affected**
Avian influenza primarily affects the respiratory and gastrointestinal systems.

**Susceptibility**
Those most susceptible to avian influenza include international travelers to visit areas where outbreaks have occurred and those who regularly come in contact with birds.

**Routes of Transmission**
Bird-to-human transmission is typically airborne.

**Signs and Symptoms**
Typical flu-like symptoms are expected, including muscle aches, fever, cough, and sore throat. However, H5N1 may also cause more severe complications, including pneumonia or acute respiratory distress.

**Patient Treatment**
Antiviral medications may be effective against H5N1, although some have proven ineffective against H5N1 strains that caused human death in Asia.

**Protective Measures**
Standard precautions and droplet precautions are indicated when caring for patients with any type of influenza virus. However, if a patient who has traveled to a country with avian influenza activity within the past 10 days presents with flu-like symptoms, precautions identical to those needed for severe acute respiratory syndrome (SARS) should be observed, including:

• Standard precautions, including thorough hand washing;
• Droplet precautions, including wearing gown and gloves for all contact;
• Airborne precautions, including using a NIOSH-approved N95 respirator; and
• Eye protection, worn anytime the caregiver is within 3 feet of the patient.

**Immunizations**
There is currently no vaccine to protect against H5N1.

| | |
|---|---|
| **Incubation Period** | There are a number of opinions regarding the incubation period in avian influenza. The expected period is 2 to 7 days. |
| **Health Care Providers** | Health care providers should be alert to any trends related to unusual flu-like activity. Early recognition, surveillance, and prevention are key to reduce the chance of a flu pandemic. |

## BOTULISM

| | |
|---|---|
| **Causative Agent** | Botulism is a type of food poisoning caused by a toxin produced by the *Clostridium botulinum* bacteria. |
| **Body Systems Affected** | Botulism affects the nervous system. |
| **Susceptibility** | Susceptibility for botulism is general. |
| **Routes of Transmission** | Transmission of botulism is through ingestion of undercooked food contaminated with the *Clostridium botulinum* bacteria. There is no evidence of person-to-person transmission of botulism. Infants are sometimes infected through the ingestion of contaminated honey. |
| **Signs and Symptoms** | Symptoms of botulism may include weakness, poor reflexes, blurred or double vision, and difficulty swallowing. Symptoms of infant botulism may include visual disturbances, poor feeding, and difficulty breathing. |
| **Patient Treatment** | Treatment for botulism is generally supportive. An antitoxin may be given in certain cases of foodborne botulism but not with infant botulism. |
| **Protective Measures** | Since botulism is not spread person to person, standard precautions should provide adequate protection. |
| **Immunizations** | There is no vaccine for botulism at this time. |
| **Incubation Period** | The incubation period for botulism may be between 12 hours and several days. The appearance of symptoms within 36 hours is not uncommon. |
| **Health Care Providers** | Since botulism is foodborne, health care providers should take care to properly cook and reheat food. Bulging cans should not be opened and honey should not be given to infants (under 1 year). |

## CANDIDIASIS

**Causative Agent**  Candidiasis is caused by an overgrowth of a normally occurring fungus called *Candida*.

**Body Systems Affected**  Candidiasis, also called yeast infection or VVC, affects the genitourinary system.

**Susceptibility**  Although men may experience candidiasis, women are more susceptible, with nearly 75% of all adult women having at least one genital yeast infection during their lifetime. Most susceptible are those who are pregnant, have diabetes mellitus, have weakened immune systems, or take corticosteroids or broad-spectrum antibiotics.

**Routes of Transmission**  Candidiasis can be transmitted through sexual intercourse; however, the most common scenario is an overgrowth of a person's own *Candida* organisms, which live in the mouth, vagina, and gastrointestinal tract. Candidiasis can also be transmitted through oral sex, from the vagina to the mouth.

**Signs and Symptoms**  Females may experience genital itching or burning and a cottage cheese–like vaginal discharge may be present. Males may experience an itchy rash on the penis.

**Patient Treatment**  Antifungal drugs, taken orally, topically, or vaginally, are drugs of choice for candidiasis.

**Protective Measures**  Standard precautions are indicated with all patients.

**Immunizations**  There is no vaccine for candidiasis at this time.

**Incubation Period**  The incubation period is thought to be 2–5 days.

**Health Care Providers**  Health care providers should consider the possibility of candidiasis even when the patient is not sexually active. Although it is considered a sexually transmitted disease (STD), candidiasis is not frequently transmitted sexually. In fact, those who have never been sexually active are also susceptible.

## CHLAMYDIA

**Causative Agent**  *Chlamydia trachomatis* is the causative agent for chlamydia.

**Body Systems Affected**  *Chlamydia* affects the eyes, genitals, and respiratory system.

| Susceptibility | Susceptibility is general. It is estimated that 25% of men may be carriers. Unlike some other diseases, it appears there is no acquired immunity for *chlamydia* after infection. |
| Routes of Transmission | *Chlamydia* is typically considered a sexually transmitted disease, although it may be transmitted by sharing contaminated clothing or towels. Infected eye secretions may be transmitted hand to hand. |
| Signs and Symptoms | Common signs and symptoms include **conjunctivitis, dysuria** and **purulent** urinary discharge. |
| Patient Treatment | Patient care is supportive. Antibiotics may be prescribed. |
| Protective Measures | Standard precautions and diligent hand washing should be practiced. |
| Immunizations | No immunization is available at this time. |
| Incubation Period | Incubation period is 1 week to 1 month. |
| Health Care Providers | Health care providers should take care in handling contaminated clothing or linens. All contaminated linen should be placed in a biohazard bag and treated as infectious. As always, good hand washing is essential. |

## CHICKENPOX

| Causative Agent | Chickenpox is caused by the varicella–zoster virus. |
| Body Systems Affected | The integumentary system is the primary body system affected. |
| Susceptibility | Susceptibility is general. |
| Routes of Transmission | Chickenpox is considered an airborne transmitted disease, although it may be transmitted by contact with items contaminated with discharges from skin lesions of an infected person. |
| Signs and Symptoms | A rash, primarily on the trunk, begins as small red spots that become blisters (Figure A-3). Once these blisters collapse, they dry into scabs. Patients also experience respiratory symptoms, generalized weakness, and low-grade fever. |
| Patient Treatment | Care is primarily supportive. **Antiviral** drugs may be helpful. |

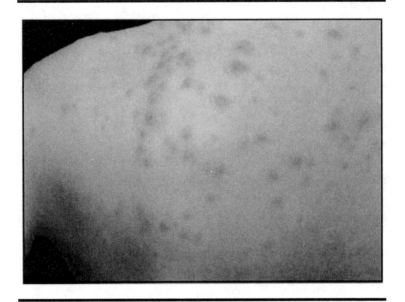

**FIGURE A-3** Chickenpox. (Photo courtesy of the Centers for Disease Control and Prevention.)

**Protective Measures**   Persons with chickenpox should avoid public places until all **lesions** are crusted and dry. Health care providers should observe standard airborne and contact precautions, take care in handling soiled linen, and wash hands thoroughly after patient contact.

**Immunizations**      A vaccine is available and recommended for unvaccinated or nonimmune health care providers. The vaccine should not be given to pregnant women or those with depressed immune systems.

**Incubation Period**   Incubation period may be between 7 and 21 days, although it is typically 14 to 17 days.

**Health Care Providers**      Health care providers who cannot prove immunity to chicken pox should take the live, **attenuated** varicella vaccine. Although there is some controversy surrounding how immunity should be proved, the CDC suggests that confirmation by a parent or other responsible adult of someone having chickenpox during childhood should be adequate to suggest immunity.

Both standard and airborne precautions should be taken and extreme care should be used in handling soiled linens. All contaminated linens should be placed in a biohazard bag.

## CLOSTRIDIUM DIFFICILE INFECTION

**Causative Agent**

*Chlostridium difficile* is a spore-forming, gram-positive bacillus that can cause diarrhea, colitis, and sepsis.

**Body Systems Affected**

*Clostridium difficile* primarily affects the intestinal system.

**Susceptibility**

Those who are elderly or have illnesses requiring prolonged use of antibiotics are at increased risk for contracting this disease.

**Routes of Transmission**

*C. difficile* is found in feces. Any item that becomes contaminated with feces may serve as a reservoir for *C. difficile* spores. Transmission is typically through contaminated hands coming in contact with the mouth or other mucous membranes.

**Signs and Symptoms**

Signs and symptoms include nausea, watery diarrhea, loss of appetite, fever, abdominal pain, and tenderness.

**Patient Treatment**

In nearly a quarter of patients, *C. difficile*–associated disease resolves itself within 2 to 3 days of discontinuing the patient's antibiotic. A 10-day course of oral vancomycin or metronidazole may be indicated.

**Protective Measures**

Standard precautions are indicated with all patients. When the patient is incontinent or the caregiver may come in contact with feces, contact precautions should also be taken.

**Immunizations**

There is no vaccine for *C. difficile*.

**Incubation Period**

The exact incubation period is unknown, although it is thought to be less than 1 week.

**Health Care Providers**

The spread of C. *difficile* should prompt health care providers to:

- Use antibiotics judiciously.
- Use contact precautions for patients with C. *difficile*–associated disease.
- Perform thorough hand washing with soap and water or an alcohol hand rub.
- Use gloves during patient care.
- Use gowns if soiling of clothing is likely.
- Implement a disinfecting environmental cleaning strategy that includes adequate cleaning of environmental surfaces and using an Environmental Protection Agency (EPA)–registered hypochorlite-based disinfectant.

# CRYPTOSPORIDIOSIS

**Causative Agent**

The causative agent of cryptosporidiosis is cryptosporidium, a single-celled parasitic protozoan that lives in the intestines of people and animals. The **dormant** (inactive) form is the **oocyst**, which is excreted from the feces of infected humans and animals. The oocyst is **environmentally resistant** and can survive outside of the body for long periods of time.

**Body Systems Affected**

The primary body system affected by cryptosporidiosis is the gastrointestinal (GI) system.

**Susceptibility**

Susceptibility is general, although those with weakened immune systems tend to have more severe symptoms. Anyone who consumes contaminated food or water or is exposed to the fecal material of an infected person may be at risk. Entire municipal water systems have been affected. Outbreaks of cryptosporidiosis have been documented in Carrollton, Georgia, and Milwaukee, Wisconsin. In Milwaukee, an estimated 400,000 people became ill during a single outbreak. Additional outbreaks have been documented at day care centers.

**Routes of Transmission**

This disease is basically waterborne, although it may be transmitted person to person through exposure to the feces of an infected person.

| | |
|---|---|
| **Signs and Symptoms** | Signs and symptoms include watery diarrhea, abdominal cramps, fever, dehydration, weight loss, and nausea. |
| **Patient Treatment** | Treatment is supportive. Persons who are dehydrated or susceptible to dehydration may need intravenous fluid therapy. |
| **Protective Measures** | Standard precautions should be taken with all patients. In addition, contact precautions should be taken and hand washing should be meticulous. |
| **Immunizations** | There is no immunization available at this time. |
| **Incubation Period** | Incubation period typically is between 2 and 10 days, although the average is 7 days. |
| **Health Care Providers** | Health care providers should remember that oocysts are not killed with typical disinfectants. Heat of 160°F is necessary to kill the protozoa. Good hand washing, standard precautions, and care in handling soiled linens and equipment should be taken. |

## CYTOMEGALOVIRUS (CMV)

| | |
|---|---|
| **Causative Agent** | The causative agent of CMV is cytomegalovirus, a member of the herpesvirus group. Although it is very common, CMV rarely causes illness and often goes undetected. |
| **Body Systems Affected** | In the average person, CMV will cause no significant effects. However, in the immunocompromised patient, the eyes may be affected. Persons with AIDS may experience retinal infections that could lead to blindness. |
| **Susceptibility** | Susceptibility is general, in that anyone may become infected. However, CMV infection is more likely in developing countries and in areas with low socioeconomic conditions. Risks are also greater for unborn babies and newborns as well as for those who are immunocompromised. |
| **Routes of Transmission** | CMV infection is typically transmitted through urine, saliva, blood, semen, tears, or breast milk of an infected person. Person-to-person transmission usually takes place when infected body fluid comes |

in contact with the hands and the hands spread the infection to the mouth or nose. It can also be sexually transmitted.

**Signs and Symptoms**   Although CMV seldom causes illness, when signs and symptoms occur they may appear similar to those seen with infectious mononucleosis. Signs such as fatigue, malaise, fever, chills, and muscle aches may be expected. Immunocompromised persons and those who have received organ transplants may experience more dangerous symptoms, including infections of the retina and blindness.

**Patient Treatment**   Most persons with CMV do not require treatment. Treatment, when indicated, is supportive. Pharmacological therapy using ganciclovir and foscarnet may be helpful in the immunocompromised patient, although they are not recommended for the otherwise healthy patient because of the sometimes severe side effects they may cause.

**Protective Measures**   Standard precautions and good hand washing should be observed. Use care when handling contaminated linens, equipment, and personal effects of infected patients, as the virus may be active on these surfaces.

**Immunizations**   An immunization for CMV is in the early stages of development, but is not yet available.

**Incubation Period**   The typical incubation period is 20 to 60 days, although it may be shorter in the immunocompromised patient.

**Health Care Providers**   Health care providers should observe standard precautions and good hand washing. Limit exposure to personal items and place exposed linens in a biohazard bag. Decontaminate all affected equipment.

## ESCHERICHIA COLI (DIARRHEAGENIC OR NON-SHIGA TOXIN-PRODUCING)

**Causative Agent**   A variety of *Escherichia coli* serotypes can cause *E. coli*. Four major groups include: **enterotoxigenic (ETEC)**, **enteroaggregative (EAgg EC)**, **enteroinvasive (EIEC)**, and **enteropathogenic (EPEC)**.

| | |
|---|---|
| **Body Systems Affected** | *E. coli* affects the gastrointestinal system. |
| **Susceptibility** | Those most susceptible to *E. coli* are international travelers. EPEC and EIEC are most common among young children in developing countries, whereas those who are immunocompromised are susceptible to EAggEC. |
| **Routes of Transmission** | Although person-to-person transmission is possible, most are exposed to *E. coli* by ingestion of food or water contaminated with human or animal feces. |
| **Signs and Symptoms** | Those who contract *E. coli* may have fever, and usually have watery or bloody diarrhea and abdominal cramps. |
| **Patient Treatment** | Treatment is focused on maintaining hydration. Other specific treatments may be applicable, depending on the type of *E. coli*. |
| **Protective Measures** | Standard and contact precautions should be taken. |
| **Immunizations** | There is no vaccine to protect against *E. coli*, although some are being developed. |
| **Incubation Period** | The incubation period varies, but is usually 24 to 72 hours. |
| **Health Care Providers** | Standard precautions and thorough hand washing are in order. |

## *ESCHERICHIA COLI* (*E. COLI* O157:H7)

| | |
|---|---|
| **Causative Agent** | *Escherichia coli* are bacteria normally found in the intestines of humans and animals. Most strains of *E. coli* are harmless, but *E. coli* O157:H7, a member of the **enterohemorrhagic** group, can cause severe illness. |
| **Body Systems Affected** | *E. coli* O157:H7 affects the gastrointestinal system and the kidneys. |
| **Susceptibility** | Susceptibility for *E. coli* is general. |
| **Routes of Transmission** | Transmission is primarily foodborne, caused by eating undercooked meat containing the bacteria. However, person-to-person transmission can take place when bacteria from diarrheal stools of infected persons are spread through inadequate hygiene and/or hand washing. |

| | |
|---|---|
| **Signs and Symptoms** | The most common symptoms are diarrhea (sometimes bloody), and abdominal cramps, which last 5 to 10 days. In severe cases, the infection can cause **hemolytic–uremic syndrome**, in which red blood cells are destroyed and kidneys eventually fail. |
| **Patient Treatment** | Care is supportive and may include fluid replacement to combat dehydration. |
| **Protective Measures** | Standard precautions should be observed, along with good hand washing. When the patient is incontinent, contact precautions should be taken. |
| **Immunizations** | There is no vaccination for *E. coli* at this time. |
| **Incubation Period** | Symptoms usually appear in about 3 days, though the range may be 1 to 9 days. |
| **Health Care Providers** | Health care providers should observe standard precautions and good hand washing practices. Avoid handling fecal material and place all contaminated materials in biohazard bags. |

## GONORRHEA

| | |
|---|---|
| **Causative Agent** | *Neisseria gonorrhea* is the causative agent for gonorrhea. |
| **Body Systems Affected** | Gonorrhea typically affects genital organs and associated structures. |
| **Susceptibility** | Susceptibility is general but targeted to those who have unprotected sexual intercourse with infected persons. After exposure, antibodies develop, but only for the specific strain of gonorrhea involved. Those who have been previously exposed may be at greater risk for infection by another strain. |
| **Routes of Transmission** | Transmission is through direct contact with **exudates** of mucous membranes and almost always occurs through unprotected sexual intercourse. |
| **Signs and Symptoms** | Males typically report an inflammation of the urethra with associated dysuria and purulent urinary discharge. If untreated, this can progress to **epididymitis, prostatitis,** and **urethral strictures.** |
| | Females typically report dysuria with a purulent vaginal discharge. Untreated, gonorrhea may progress to **pelvic inflammatory disease (PID),** |

causing lower abdominal pain, fever, and abnormal menstrual bleeding. Menstruation gives bacteria the opportunity to spread from the cervix to the upper genital tract, and causes 50% of PID cases occurring within 1 week of the onset of menstruation. Gonorrhea puts females at increased risk of ectopic pregnancy; sterility; and abscesses of the ovaries, fallopian tubes, and other reproductive structures. In rare cases, a **systemic bacteremia** may occur, causing **septic arthritis** with swelling of the joints accompanied by fever and pain. If left untreated, progressive deterioration of the joints may occur.

**Patient Treatment**

Initial treatment is supportive. Antibiotics may be indicated.

**Protective Measures**

Standard precautions and good hand washing are essential. Place affected linens in biohazard bags and decontaminate exposed equipment.

**Immunizations**

There is no vaccine available for gonorrhea at this time.

**Incubation Period**

Average incubation period is 3 to 7 days, although it may range from a low of 2 days to a high of 30 days.

**Health Care Providers**

Health care providers should use extreme caution when handling soiled linen and should consider any body fluid as potentially infectious.

# HANTAVIRUS PULMONARY SYNDROME

**Causative Agent**

Hantavirus is the causative agent.

**Body Systems Affected**

Hantavirus pulmonary syndrome, as its name suggests, eventually affects the respiratory system. The musculoskeletal system may also be affected.

**Susceptibility**

Susceptibility is general. Persons who live or work in areas where rodents or rodent droppings may be found are more likely to be exposed.

**Routes of Transmission**

It is thought that hantavirus is spread when humans inhale microscopic particles that contain rodent droppings or urine.

**Signs and Symptoms**

Persons with hantavirus pulmonary syndrome may be expected to report muscle aches, headaches, and coughs. A high fever may also occur. After a few days respiratory symptoms may develop, which may grow into pulmonary edema and eventually, respiratory failure.

**Patient Treatment**

Treatment is primarily supportive. Some physicians have used ribavarin in an attempt to treat the disease.

**Protective Measures**

This disease is not considered person-to-person transmissible. Standard precautions are indicated when caring for a patient with hantavirus pulmonary syndrome. However, when working in rodent-infested areas, the health care provider should wear eye and respiratory protection and should avoid contact with rodents and their droppings.

**Immunizations**

There is no vaccine for hantavirus pulmonary syndrome at this time.

**Incubation Period**

The incubation period may range from a few days to 6 weeks. Typical incubation period is 1 to 2 weeks.

**Health Care Providers**

Health care providers should use caution any time they are exposed to an area infested by rodents. Masks, eye protection, and gloves are indicated to protect oneself from the disease-causing agent.

## HEPATITIS A

**Causative Agent**

Hepatitis A is caused by the hepatitis A virus.

**Body Systems Affected**

All forms of hepatitis affect the liver.

**Susceptibility**

Susceptibility is general in that there is no clearly defined population at increased risk of hepatitis A. However, those with potential for exposure to fecal material are more likely to be exposed.

**Routes of Transmission**

Hepatitis A may be transmitted person to person through the fecal–oral route. Since hepatitis A can survive on unwashed hands for up to 4 hours, day care workers should be careful to observe good hand washing practices. It may also be transmitted through contaminated water or food, and in some cases may be transmitted through sexual or household contact.

**Signs and Symptoms**   Many infected persons are asymptomatic. Those who experience symptoms may report right upper quadrant abdominal pain, anorexia, nausea, fever, and weakness. Symptoms are typically mild in severity and last no more than 6 weeks.

**Patient Treatment**   Care is supportive, with an emphasis on treating the symptoms.

**Protective Measures**   Standard precautions and good hand washing should be the rule with all patients. Contact precautions should be taken to isolate the caregiver from contact with fecal material.

**Immunizations**   An inactivated hepatitis A vaccine is available. The CDC suggests that immunization against hepatitis A may be indicated for health care workers.

**Incubation Period**   The incubation period is typically 2 to 6 weeks.

**Health Care Providers**   Health care providers should take standard precautions and should practice good hand washing habits. Immunization against hepatitis A should be considered.

## HEPATITIS B

**Causative Agent**   Hepatitis B virus is the causative agent.

**Body Systems Affected**   Hepatitis B affects the liver and may cause **necrosis**.

**Susceptibility**   Susceptibility is general, although those with exposure to infected blood or blood-containing body fluids are at greater risk.

**Routes of Transmission**   Blood, semen, vaginal fluids, and saliva may all be considered infectious. Hepatitis B may be transmitted through exposure to blood and blood-containing body fluid through occupational exposure, sexual contact, or contact with contaminated needles.

**Signs and Symptoms**   Persons infected with hepatitis B typically report cold and flu-like symptoms, including fever, joint pain, general weakness, anorexia, and nausea and vomiting. Since the disease affects the liver, jaundice may occur.

**Patient Treatment**   Care for the patient with hepatitis B is primarily supportive.

**Protective Measures**   Standard precautions are essential, as is effective hand washing.

**Immunizations**

Recombinant vaccines (Recombivax HB and Engerix B) are available and given in a series of three intramuscular injections. The first dose is followed in 1 month by a second dose. The third, and final, dose is given 6 months after the initial dose. For more information on the hepatitis B vaccine, see Chapter 5.

**Incubation Period**   The incubation period for hepatitis B is typically 1 to 6 months, although it may be as long as 200 days.

**Health Care Providers**

Hepatitis B is environmentally resistant, which means the virus can survive outside the body for long periods of time. Because of this, health care providers should use extreme caution when dealing with any blood or blood-containing body fluid. Standard precautions and good hand washing techniques are essential, as are proper disposal of contaminated linens, equipment, and supplies. Experts tell us that the environmental resistance of hepatitis B makes it 200 times easier to become infected with HBV than with HIV.

# HEPATITIS C

**Causative Agent**   The causative agent is the hepatitis C virus.

**Body Systems Affected**   Hepatitis C primarily affects the liver.

**Susceptibility**   Susceptibility to hepatitic C virus is greater for health care providers than for the general population. When exposed to blood containing the virus, health care providers experience a 2.7 to 10% probability of contracting the infection. Probability of contracting the disease through household or sexual contact is lower. Hepatitis C is not known to be transmitted through contaminated food or water.

**Routes of Transmission**   Hepatitis C is transmitted through blood or blood-containing body fluid. Typical routes of transmission are through needlesticks or accidental exposure to blood or blood-containing body fluids.

Exposure may be through splashes into the mucous membranes around the eyes, nose, or mouth or through blood coming in contact with nonintact skin.

**Signs and Symptoms**

When symptoms are present, they typically mimic the symptoms of the flu. Often there are no symptoms, so by the time a person finds out he/she has hepatitis C, there may already be serious liver damage.

**Patient Treatment**

Treatment is supportive, although an extensive regimen of pharmacologic therapy is available. This 48-week course of antiviral drugs suppresses the virus in 41% of those who test positive for the disease.

**Protective Measures**

Standard precautions and effective hand washing are essential.

**Immunizations**

Although a vaccine is currently under development, no immunization is currently available.

**Incubation Period**

The incubation period may range between 2 and 26 weeks, although the average incubation period is 6 to 8 weeks.

**Health Care Providers**

Health care providers who are expected to have occupational exposure to blood and other potentially infectious material are at risk for becoming infected with the hepatitis C virus. Thousands of health care providers who did not use personal protective equipment and standard precautions in the 1970s and 1980s have contracted the disease. Since many infected persons are asymptomatic, severe liver damage can occur before learning of the infection.

## HEPATITIS NON-ABC

**Causative Agent**

The primary viruses responsible for non-ABC hepatitis include hepatitis D (delta) virus; hepatitis E, which is similar to hepatitis A; and hepatitis G, which is a newly identified virus.

**Body Systems Affected**

As with all strains of hepatitis, non-ABC hepatitis viruses affect the liver.

**Susceptibility**

Susceptibility is general, although it should be noted that the hepatitis D virus requires the presence of hepatitis B to **replicate**. When the hepatitis D virus becomes active in people infected with hepatitis B, the resulting disease becomes extremely **pathogenic**.

**Routes of Transmission**    Hepatitis D and G are bloodborne, whereas hepatitis E is transmitted through exposure to infected fecal matter.

**Signs and Symptoms**    The onset of hepatitis D is abrupt, with signs and symptoms mimicking the hepatitis B virus. It is always associated with, and often mistaken for, hepatitis B. Many patients with hepatitis E are asymptomatic. Symptoms, when they occur, include nausea, fever, abdominal pain, and generalized weakness.

**Patient Treatment**    Care is supportive.

**Protective Measures**    Standard precautions and effective hand washing are essential.

**Immunizations**    Hepatitis B vaccine can indirectly prevent hepatitis D but has no effect on hepatitis E. Immunity to hepatitis B equates to immunity to hepatitis D.

**Incubation Period**    The incubation period of hepatitis D is 21 to 90 days. The hepatitis E incubation period may range from 15 to 60 days, but 40 days is the average. The incubation period of hepatitis G is not yet known.

**Health Care Providers**    Although there is still much to be learned about hepatitis non-ABC, health care providers should take standard precautions with all patients and stay abreast of emerging developments with regard to these diseases.

## HERPES SIMPLEX TYPE 1

**Causative Agent**    Herpes simplex type 1 is caused by the herpes simplex virus type 1 (HSV-1).

**Body Systems Affected**    Herpes simplex type 1 affects the oropharnyx, face, lips, skin, fingers, toes, and, in infants, the central nervous system and may be passed to the genitalia via the hands.

**Susceptibility**    Susceptibility is general.

**Routes of Transmission**    Herpes simplex virus is typically transmitted through saliva and infection on the hands.

| | |
|---|---|
| **Signs and Symptoms** | Patients will likely experience cold sores and fever blisters, generally found on the lips, face, conjuctiva, or oropharnyx. |
| **Patient Treatment** | Care is supportive. Pharmacological therapy with acyclovir (Zovirax) is available. Acyclovir, which may be taken orally or topically, prevents the virus from replicating, but will not eradicate it. |
| **Protective Measures** | Standard precautions are indicated. |
| **Immunizations** | No vaccine is available at this time. |
| **Incubation Period** | The incubation period of herpes simplex 1 is not yet known. |
| **Health Care Providers** | Since lesions are highly contagious, health care providers should take care to use standard precautions. |

## HERPES SIMPLEX TYPE 2 (GENITAL HERPES)

| | |
|---|---|
| **Causative Agent** | Herpes simplex virus type 2 (HSV-2) is the causative agent for genital herpes. |
| **Body Systems Affected** | Body regions affected include those regions associated with intimate sexual contact. |
| **Susceptibility** | Susceptibility is general. |
| **Routes of Transmission** | Transmission is through sexual intercourse. |
| **Signs and Symptoms** | Males report painful lesions on the penis, anus, rectum, and/or mouth, depending on the sexual practices of the affected person. |
| | Females are sometimes asymptomatic but may report lesions on the anus, rectum, vulva, cervix, or mouth, depending on the sexual practices of the affected person. Recurrences generally affect the buttocks, legs, perineal skin, and vulva. |
| **Patient Treatment** | Care is supportive. Pharmacological therapy with acyclovir (Zovirax) may be helpful in preventing the virus from replicating, but will not eradicate it. Acyclovir is available in both oral and topical forms. |
| **Protective Measures** | Standard precautions are recommended and especially important when handling affected linen and supplies. |
| **Immunizations** | There is no vaccine for genital herpes at this time. |

| | |
|---|---|
| **Incubation Period** | The incubation period for herpes simplex type 2 is not yet known. |
| **Health Care Providers** | Health care providers should use extreme caution when handling linen or equipment exposed to the affected area(s). Standard precautions and effective hand washing are the best lines of defense for the health care provider. |

## INFLUENZA

| | |
|---|---|
| **Causative Agent** | Influenza results from influenza virus types A, B, and C. |
| **Body Systems Affected** | Influenza primarily affects the respiratory system. |
| **Susceptibility** | Susceptibility is general. Persons at greatest risk of influenza are those who have the greatest opportunity for exposure and those who have weakened immune systems. |
| **Routes of Transmission** | Influenza is spread by inhaling droplets from a sneeze or cough, or by touching an object exposed to the influenza virus then touching the mouth, nose, or mucous membranes around the eyes. |
| **Signs and Symptoms** | Symptoms include fever, chills, headache, muscle aches, sore throat, and a severe and protracted cough. |
| **Patient Treatment** | Patient care is supportive and is aimed at making the symptoms more tolerable. |
| **Protective Measures** | Standard and droplet precautions should be taken. |
| **Immunizations**  | Immunizations are widely available and are recommended for persons over 65 years of age, residents of long-term-care facilities, persons with chronic medical conditions, persons with serious health conditions, anyone with a weakened immune system, and health care providers. Protection develops approximately 2 weeks after vaccination and lasts approximately 1 year. |
| **Incubation Period** | The incubation period is typically 1 to 3 days. |
| **Health Care Providers**  | Since health care providers are likely to come in contact with persons who have the influenza virus, they should consider taking the influenza vaccine and should always observe standard precautions and wash their hands after contact with each patient. |

## LEGIONELLOSIS

**Causative Agent**

Legionellosis is caused by the *Legionella pneumophila*. This particular bacteria was named after an outbreak among people attending an American Legion convention in 1976.

**Body Systems Affected**

Since legionellosis typically causes a bacterial pneumonia, the respiratory system is the primary system affected.

**Susceptibility**

Although susceptibility is general, the disease most often affects middle-aged or older men, especially those who drink alcohol or smoke heavily, and persons with preexisting medical conditions.

**Routes of Transmission**

Since *Legionella* bacteria grow best in warm water, people usually become infected when they breathe mist or vapor that has been contaminated with the bacteria. Examples of this type of transmission include breathing the steam from a whirlpool spa or inhaling aerosol from sources such as air-handling systems of large buildings and water used for drinking and bathing. There is no evidence that person-to-person transmission occurs.

**Signs and Symptoms**

Patients typically exhibit flu-like symptoms including muscle aches, headache, fever, chills, and diarrhea.

**Patient Treatment**

Immediate care is supportive. Antibiotics may be helpful in treating the disease.

**Protective Measures**

Since there is no evidence to support the belief that legionellosis can be spread person to person, standard precautions are all that is recommended. *Legionella* may be found in institutional water systems, ponds and creeks, and in the water in air-conditioning units.

**Immunizations**

There is currently no vaccine for legionellosis.

**Incubation Period**

Signs and symptoms typically occur within 5 to 6 days, although a range of 2 to 10 days has been recorded.

**Health Care Providers**

Since legionellosis is not transmitted person-to-person, standard precautions should be adequate protection. This disease occurs sporadically and in outbreaks.

## LICE (PEDICULOSIS AND PHTHIRIASIS)

**Causative Agent**  Three types of lice are discussed here: *Pediculosis humanus capitis* (head louse), *Pediculosis humanus corporis* (body louse), and *Phthirus pubis* (crab louse).

**Body Systems Affected**  All three types of lice affect the skin and hair (Figure A-4).

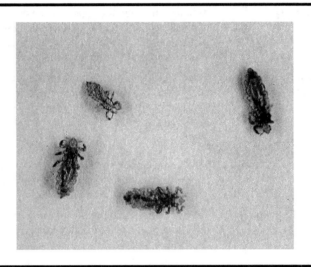

**FIGURE A-4** Detail of head lice.

**Susceptibility**  Susceptibility is general.

**Routes of Transmission**  Head lice are spread through direct contact with an infested person and/or objects used by him or her. Body lice may be spread through indirect contact with personal belongings of an infested person, especially shared clothing and headwear. Crab lice are spread through sexual contact.

**Signs and Symptoms**  The primary symptom is itching at the affected area. Head lice typically infest head and facial hair. Body lice typically infest the inner seams of clothing. Crab lice infest the genital area.

**Patient Treatment**  A **pediculicide** should be used at time of diagnosis and repeated 7 days later. Careful attention to removing all nits, or eggs, attached to the hair shaft is necessary. Vinegar and water may be used to loosen the nits prior to combing with a specialized, fine-toothed comb called a delousing comb.

**Protective Measures**

Standard precautions and thorough hand washing should be used. Linen should be bagged and the area sprayed with an insecticide known to be effective for lice and mites. Care should be taken to clean and remove insecticide residues. Contact precautions should be taken for 24 hours post treatment.

**Immunizations**

There is no vaccine for lice at this time.

**Incubation Period**

An adult louse can produce approximately six eggs every 24 hours. Eggs hatch in 7 to 10 days. Depending on the temperature, the **nymph** stage lasts 7 to 13 days. The egg-to-egg cycle lasts about 3 weeks.

**Health Care Providers**

Health care providers should remain alert to the presence of lice on their patients and check themselves thoroughly after contact with those known or believed to be infested with lice. Careful attention to checking for lice and/or nits is suggested.

# LISTERIOSIS

**Causative Agent**

Listeriosis is a bacterial infection caused by the *Listeria* bacteria. One of the most common types is *Listeria monocytogenes*. One trait of *L. monocytogenes* is that it will grow at refrigeration temperatures and will survive pasteurization and heat treatment. Freezing has little effect on the bacteria. *L. monocytogenes* is often found in soil and water.

**Body Systems Affected**

Listeriosis can cause flu-like symptoms and affect the gastrointestinal and nervous systems.

**Susceptibility**

People with weakened immune systems, pregnant women, elderly persons, and those with preexisting medical conditions are more susceptible to listeriosis than the general population.

**Routes of Transmission**

Listeriosis is typically transmitted through contaminated food, but may be transmitted to a fetus through the placenta of an infected pregnant woman.

| | |
|---|---|
| **Signs and Symptoms** | Patients with listeriosis experience flu-like symptoms, including fever, chills, nausea, vomiting, and diarrhea. Other symptoms include headache, stiff neck, upset stomach, confusion, and convulsions. |
| **Patient Treatment** | Care is mostly supportive, concentrating on the symptoms. Listeriosis may be treated with antibiotics. |
| **Protective Measures** | Since listeriosis is transmitted via contaminated food, risk of person-to-person transmission during patient care would not be expected. Standard precautions and hand washing are indicated, as with any patient. |
| **Immunizations** | There is currently no vaccine for listeriosis. |
| **Incubation Period** | The time from exposure to major symptoms can vary from a few days to approximately 3 weeks, although gastrointestinal symptoms may begin much sooner. |
| **Health Care Providers** | Listeriosis is not considered a great threat to health care providers. |

## LYME DISEASE

| | |
|---|---|
| **Causative Agent** | Lyme disease is caused by *Borrelia burgdorferi*. |
| **Body Systems Affected** | The skin, musculoskeletal system (especially the joints), central nervous system, and cardiovascular system may be affected by Lyme disease. |
| **Susceptibility** | Susceptibility for Lyme disease is general, although persons in areas of high tick infestations have more opportunity for exposure. |
| **Routes of Transmission** | Lyme disease is a tickborne disease. Major reservoirs are mice and deer. |
| **Signs and Symptoms** | Symptoms of Lyme disease occur in phases. First, a painless skin lesion at the site of the bite appears, followed quickly by flu-like symptoms, with weakness, stiff neck, and **myalgia**. Later, multiple skin lesions appear and nervous system symptoms (including meningitis, **peripheral neuropathy**, and **Bell's palsy**) commence. Cardiovascular symptoms, including myocarditis, left ventricular block, and atrioventricular block are possible, |

although the latter is more common. In later stages, chronic arthritis, depression, and sleep disorders can develop.

**Patient Treatment**

Patient treatment is supportive. Antibiotic therapy may be indicated.

**Protective Measures**

There is no evidence of person-to-person transmission of Lyme disease. However, health care providers should be alert to the presence of ticks that may be on the patient's clothing or body.

**Immunizations**

Although a commercially available vaccine was introduced in 1998, it has since been discontinued because of low sales.

**Incubation Period**

The incubation period for Lyme disease varies between 3 and 32 days.

**Health Care Providers**

Out-of-hospital health care providers, especially those who work in wilderness areas, should be aware of the presence of ticks.

## MEASLES (RUBEOLA, HARD MEASLES)

**Causative Agent**

Measles is caused by the measles virus, of the genus *Morbilli*.

**Body Systems Affected**

Measles affects the respiratory, integumentary, and central nervous systems, as well as the eyes.

**Susceptibility**

Although measles is considered a childhood disease, susceptibility is general.

**Routes of Transmission**

Measles may be spread by direct contact with nasal or throat secretions of infected persons. It can also be transmitted by airborne transmission.

**Signs and Symptoms**

Symptoms of measles typically appear in two stages. During the first stage, the patient may have a slight fever, runny nose, conjuctivitis, **photophobia**, malaise, and cough. A day or two before the generalized rash so commonly associated with measles appears, **Koplik's spots** may develop inside the mouth. The generalized rash is red, slightly bumpy, and spreads from the head and face to the lower extremities within about 3 days and disappears within about 6 days. Pneumonia, eye damage, and myocarditis develop in some patients.

**Patient Treatment**
There is no specific treatment for measles. Care is aimed at minimizing symptoms.

**Protective Measures**
Health care providers should observe standard precautions, airborne precautions, and good hand washing techniques.

**Immunizations**
An immunization against measles is available.

**Incubation Period**
Symptoms usually appear within 10 to 12 days of exposure, although a range of 8 to 13 days is possible.

**Health Care Providers**

Since measles is one of the most highly contagious infectious diseases, health care providers should ensure their immunity. In general, one may be considered immune if he/she meets one or more of the following criteria:

• has received at least one dose of live measles vaccine after first birthday
• has documentation of prior physician-diagnosed measles
• has had laboratory testing that indicates immunity
• was born before 1957

## MENINGOCOCCAL MENINGITIS

**Causative Agent**
Meningitis may be bacterial, viral, or fungal. Meningococcal (spinal) meningitis is caused by *Neisseria meningitidis* bacteria.

**Body Systems Affected**
Meningitis affects the respiratory and central nervous systems.

**Susceptibility**
Susceptibility to meningitis is general, although it has been suggested that children under 5 years, teenagers, young adults, and older people are at greater risk.

**Routes of Transmission**
Transmission is by direct contact with a patient's respiratory secretions or through airborne transmission

of respiratory droplets. The bacteria does not survive very long outside the body.

**Signs and Symptoms**

Onset is rapid. Symptoms include headache, fever, chills, vomiting, neck stiffness, joint pain, **nuchal rigidity**, and **petechial rash**. Septic shock develops in some patients.

**Patient Treatment**

Care is primarily supportive. Pharmacologic therapy with rifampin, spiramycin, minocycline, ceftriaxone, or ciprofloxacin may be indicated.

**Protective Measures**

Standard and droplet precautions are indicated, including masking both the caregiver and patient if feasible. Effective hand washing is important.

**Immunizations**

Vaccines are available that are effective against several strains of meningitis.

**Incubation Period**

Patients can carry the bacteria for days, weeks, or months before symptoms appear.

**Health Care Providers**

Health care providers should be alert to the possibility of direct transmission through contaminated linen and airway equipment. Both standard and droplet precautions are necessary.

# METHICILLIN-RESISTANT *STAPHYLOCOCCUS AUREUS* (MRSA)

**Causative Agent**

MRSA is caused by a bacteria, *Staphylococcus aureus*, that is resistant to many antibiotics. *Staph. aureus* is normally found on the skin and in the noses of healthy people.

**Body Systems Affected**

MRSA can affect a number of body systems, depending on the part of the body that is infected.

**Susceptibility**

Anyone can get MRSA, although hospitalized patients are generally more susceptible.

**Routes of Transmission**

MRSA is typically spread through direct contact with the hands of a health care provider or someone who is infected or carrying the organism.

**Signs and Symptoms**

Signs and symptoms are consistent with those of any infection. Since MRSA may affect surgical wounds, catheter sites, blood, and skin, signs and symptoms will vary depending on the part of the body that is infected.

**Patient Treatment**  Although MRSA cannot be effectively treated with methicillin, penicillin, nafcillin, and cephalosporin, other antibiotics, such as vancomycin, may be helpful.

**Protective Measures**  Standard precautions, including wearing gloves, should be taken with all patients. Contact precautions should be observed when a patient is incontinent, and a gown should be worn when there is a risk of soiling clothing. Most of all, thorough hand washing with soap and water or an alcohol-based rub is essential.

**Immunizations**  There is no vaccination for MRSA.

**Incubation Period**  The incubation period for MRSA varies.

**Health Care Providers**  It is incumbent upon health care providers to thoroughly wash their hands, to observe standard and contact precautions, and to actively work to reduce the number of hospital-associated infections.

# MONONUCLEOSIS

**Causative Agent**  Mononucleosis is a viral disease caused by the Epstein–Barr virus. It affects certain types of white blood cells.

**Body Systems Affected**  Mononucleosis affects the oropharnyx, tonsils, and respiratory system.

**Susceptibility**  Susceptibility is general. Prior infection by Epstein–Barr virus generally confers a high degree of resistance.

**Routes of Transmission**  Transmission of mononucleosis is person to person via saliva. In rare instances, mononucleosis has been transmitted by blood transfusion.

**Signs and Symptoms**  Symptoms of mononucleosis include sore throat, fever, swollen glands, and fatigue. Sometimes the liver and spleen are affected.

**Patient Treatment**  Treatment for mononucleosis is primarily supportive, with an emphasis on rest and drinking plenty of fluids. **Nonsteroidal antiinflammatory drugs (NSAIDs)** may be of value in relief of symptoms.

**Protective Measures**   Health care providers should follow good hand washing techniques and observe standard precautions.

**Immunizations**   There is no vaccine for mononucleosis.

**Incubation Period**   Symptoms of mononucleosis typically appear 4 to 6 weeks after exposure.

**Health Care Providers**   Since the virus may be active in the patient's throat for as long as 1 year after infection, health care providers should be alert to the possibility of infection through direct contact with infected saliva. For this reason, health care providers should observe standard precautions and good hand washing techniques.

## MUMPS

**Causative Agent**   Mumps is a very contagious viral disease caused by the mumps virus, of the genus *Paramyxovirus*.

**Body Systems Affected**   Mumps affects the salivary glands and may affect the central nervous system.

**Susceptibility**   Susceptibility is general. Before the mumps vaccine became widely available, nearly every child caught mumps. The vaccine is widely available today, and those who do not take it are at risk of contracting the disease.

**Routes of Transmission**   Mumps is spread person to person through direct contact with infected saliva and through droplets from a cough or sneeze.

**Signs and Symptoms**   Approximately one third of patients with mumps experience no symptoms. Those with symptoms report severe swelling and soreness of the salivary glands in cheeks and jaw, neck or ear pain, headache, tiredness, and fever.

**Patient Treatment**   Care of patients with mumps is supportive. Emphasis should be placed on pushing oral fluids and bed rest. NSAIDs may be taken to control fever. Warm moist towels may be placed to relieve swelling and pain.

**Protective Measures**   Standard precautions, droplet precautions, and effective hand washing are essential.

| | |
|---|---|
| **Immunizations**  | A mumps vaccine is readily available and should be taken by adults born after 1956 who have no proof of immunity, health care providers, and susceptible adolescents and adults who travel abroad. |
| **Incubation Period** | Symptoms usually appear between 12 and 25 days after exposure. |
| **Health Care Providers** | Since infected health care providers may spread the virus to patients, they should make sure they are immune to the disease and should take care to decontaminate infected equipment and supplies after use on a patient with mumps. |

## PERTUSSIS (WHOOPING COUGH)

| | |
|---|---|
| **Causative Agent** | Pertussis is a highly contagious bacterial infection caused by *Bordetella pertussis.* |
| **Body Systems Affected** | Pertussis affects the oropharynx and respiratory tract. |
| **Susceptibility** | Anyone exposed to the disease can be infected by pertussis. Previous infection generally confers immunity, although subsequent attacks in adolescents and adults suggests that immunity may decrease over time. |
| **Routes of Transmission** | Pertussis is spread by direct contact with respiratory discharges or through exposure to airborne droplets from a cough. |
| **Signs and Symptoms** | Initially, symptoms mimic those of the common cold, and include sneezing, runny nose, cough, and mild fever. This is called the catarrhal stage. Within 2 weeks, the cough becomes severe and is characterized by episodes of repeated rapid coughs followed by a crowing or high-pitched whoop. It is during this paroxysmal stage that pertussis is typically diagnosed. The whoop may not be present in infants under 6 months and in adults. Thick clear mucus may be discharged. Symptoms may continue for 1 to 2 months and will typically be milder in older adults. Recovery is gradual. During the last, or convalescent, stage |

the cough becomes less paroxysmal and disappears over 2 to 3 weeks.

**Patient Treatment**  Care is primarily supportive. Antibiotics, including erythromycin, may be helpful in decreasing the period of communicability.

**Protective Measures**  Caregivers should take standard precautions and droplet precautions and practice thorough hand washing techniques. Care should be taken when handling linens contaminated with respiratory secretions.

**Immunizations**  A vaccination against pertussis is included in the DTP and DtaP vaccines. Prior infection with pertussis typically confers prolonged immunity.

**Incubation Period**  The typical incubation period is 5 to 10 days, although it may be as long as 21 days.

**Health Care Providers**  Since many cases of pertussis are misdiagnosed as colds or flu, the health care provider should consistently use standard precautions and good hand washing procedures. Care should be taken in handling infected linens and respiratory equipment and supplies.

# PLAGUE

**Causative Agent**  Plague is caused by a bacterium called *Yersinia pestis* found in rodents and their fleas.

**Body Systems Affected**  Pneumonic plague affects the respiratory system, whereas bubonic plague affects the lymphatic system and, if untreated, the respiratory system.

**Susceptibility**  Persons who come in contact with plague-infested rodents are more likely to catch bubonic plague.

**Routes of Transmission**  There are two types of plague: bubonic (transmitted through the bite of an infected flea or exposure to infected material through nonintact skin) and pneumonic (transmitted person to person or through inhalation of airborne *Y. pestis* particles).

| | |
|---|---|
| **Signs and Symptoms** | Bubonic plague signs and symptoms include tender, swollen lymph glands called buboes. If untreated, bubonic plague can progress to pneumonic plague. Signs and symptoms of pneumonic plague include weakness, fever, and rapidly developing pneumonia with chest pain, cough, and shortness of breath. Watery or bloody sputum may be present, and nausea, vomiting, and abdominal pain may occur. If not treated aggressively, pneumonic plague may lead to respiratory failure, shock, and death. |
| **Patient Treatment** | Antibiotics, including doxycycline and ciprofloxacin should be given within 24 hours of the first symptoms. |
| **Protective Measures** | Standard and respiratory precautions should be taken. |
| **Immunizations** | Although research is taking place, there is currently no vaccine for plague. |
| **Incubation Period** | The incubation period of bubonic plague is typically 2 to 6 days, while the incubation period of respiratory plague is typically shorter, usually 1 to 3 days. |
| **Health Care Providers** | Since plague may be used as a biological weapon, health care providers should be aware of the signs and symptoms of pneumonic plague. |

## PNEUMONIA

| | |
|---|---|
| **Causative Agent** | Over 3 million cases of pneumonia are reported each year in the United States. Up to one third of these patients are hospitalized, which accounts for 10% of adult acute care hospital admissions in the United States. Pneumonia may be bacterial, viral, or fungal. Viral pneumonia is rare in adults except during outbreaks. Bacterial sources of pneumonia include *Streptococcus pneumoniae, Mycoplasma pneumoniae, Staphylococcus aureus, Haemophilus influenzae, Klebsiella pneumoniae, Moraxella catarrhalis,* and *Legionella* (Figure A-5). |
| **Body Systems Affected** | Pneumonia affects the respiratory and central nervous system. It may also affect the ears, nose, and throat. |

* Streptococcus pneumoniae
* Mycoplasma pneumoniae
* Staphylococcus aureus
* Haemophilus influenzae
* Klebsiella pneumoniae
* Moraxella catarrhalis
* Legionella

**FIGURE A-5** Bacterial sources of pneumonia. Pneumonia may be caused by one of many possible sources.

**Susceptibility**

Anyone exposed to the disease can catch pneumonia, although certain groups may be considered more susceptible because of decreased resistance to the disease. These groups include those who are elderly, have significant preexisting illness, or are immunocompromised.

**Routes of Transmission**

Pneumonia is spread through respiratory exposure to droplets from a sneeze or cough, or direct contact with objects contaminated with respiratory secretions of those who have pneumonia.

**Signs and Symptoms**

Persons who have pneumonia report sudden onset of chills, fever, chest discomfort, and shortness of breath. Coughs may be productive, with yellow-green phlegm. In children, be alert to high fever, tachycardia, and chest retractions, which are ominous signs.

**Patient Treatment**

Initial care is primarily supportive. Antibiotics, including erythromycin, doxycycline, augmentin, cephalosporin, and vacomycin may be used.

**Protective Measures**

Standard, airborne, and droplet precautions should be taken and hand washing after patient contact should be thorough.

**Immunizations**

A vaccine that protects against some causes of pneumonia is currently available. Although it will not protect against pneumonia of every cause, it will protect against approximately 88% of pneumococcal bacteria that cause pneumonia. Immunity is better for younger people, and the immunity lasts up to 10 years for most people.

**Incubation Period**

Most experts agree that the incubation period for pneumonia may be as short as 1 to 3 days.

**Health Care Providers**

Since health care providers are often called on to treat patients with pneumococcal disease, they should consider taking the vaccine. Standard and droplet precautions should be taken.

# RABIES

**Causative Agent**

Rabies is a viral disease of the central nervous system. The causative agent, rabies virus of the genus *Lyssavirus*, is found in domestic and wild animals.

**Body Systems Affected**

Rabies affects the central nervous system.

**Susceptibility**

Susceptibility is general for anyone who is bitten by an infected animal.

**Routes of Transmission**

Humans most frequently become infected with rabies through the virus-laden saliva from the scratch or bite of an infected animal. Person-to-person transmission is theoretically possible, although no case has been documented.

**Signs and Symptoms**

Symptoms of rabies typically present in three phases. During the **prodromal** phase, the patient presents with fever, pharyngitis, headache, anorexia, and pain, or **paresthesia**, at the site of the bite or scratch. These symptoms usually last 2 to 10 days. The second, or neurologic stage, presents with **aphasia**, paresis, paralysis, lack of coordination, mental status changes, and hyperactivity. Third-stage symptoms may include hypotension, coma, cardiac arrhythmias, **disseminated intravascular coagulation (DIC)**, cardiac arrest, and death.

Other nonspecific signs of rabies include **myoclonus**, hypersalivation, agitation, anxiety, and increased **lacrimation**.

**Patient Treatment**

Management of rabies includes thorough **debridement** of the wound, drainage as necessary, and vigorous cleaning of the wound with soap and water followed by irrigation with 70% alcohol. Human rabies immune globin (HRIG) should be administered, and patients should be immunized with human diploid cell vaccine (HDCV) or rabies vaccine. Tetanus prophylaxis and antibiotics should be administered as indicated.

**Protective Measures**

Although transmission from human patients to health care providers has never been documented, standard precautions should be used and thorough hand washing should take place.

**Immunizations**

Rabies vaccine is available as a human diploid-cell vaccine (HDCV) and an **adsorbed** vaccine (RVA). Immunization is typically directed toward individuals with high probability of exposure.

**Incubation Period**

The incubation period of rabies is usually between 3 and 8 weeks, although it may be as few as 5 days or as long as 1 year, or longer.

**Health Care Providers**

Although human-to-human transmission has not been documented, standard precautions should be taken and handwashing should be thorough. EMS workers and those who work in wilderness or other outdoor settings should be especially cautious when dealing with and working around animals. The animal source of reported rabies cases is most commonly raccoons, bats, skunks, foxes, and dogs.

## ROCKY MOUNTAIN SPOTTED FEVER

**Causative Agent**

Rocky Mountain Spotted Fever (RMSF) is caused by a specialized bacteria called *Rickettsia rickettsii*.

**Body Systems Affected**

Major complications associated with RMSF include kidney failure and shock. The liver and lungs may also be affected.

**Susceptibility**

Susceptibility is general, but those who work outdoors and have greater opportunity for exposure to ticks are more likely to be infected. RMSF has been reported throughout the United States, with the exception of Alaska, Hawaii, and Maine. Most cases are reported in the eastern United States.

**Routes of Transmission** Transmission is typically from the bite of an infected tick or by contamination of broken skin with the body fluids of a tick crushed while still attached. Person-to-person transmission is possible through transfusion of infected blood, although transmission through this route is extremely rare.

**Signs and Symptoms** Patients frequently report fever, headache, tiredness, nausea and vomiting, and deep muscle pain. The rash associated with RMSF may begin on the legs or arms, and may rapidly spread to the rest of the body. The rash initially appears as small red spots or blotches and may later change to look more like bruises or bloody patches under the skin.

**Patient Treatment** Initial treatment is supportive. Antibiotic therapy with tetracycline or chloramphenicol may be effective.

**Protective Measures** Although RMSF is not contagious person to person, standard precautions should be observed.

**Immunizations** There is no vaccine for RMSF at this time.

**Incubation Period** Symptoms of RMSF typically begin 3 to 12 days after a tick bite, although they may occur as early as 1 day or as many as 14 days after exposure.

**Health Care Providers** Although the risk of person-to-person transmission is very minor, health care providers who work in outdoor and wilderness areas should be alert to the possibility of ticks and should check themselves for ticks frequently, use insect repellents, and dress appropriately for the environment for maximal tick protection.

# RUBELLA (GERMAN MEASLES)

**Causative Agent** Rubella is an infectious disease caused by the rubella virus.

**Body Systems Affected** Rubella affects the respiratory, integumentary, musculoskeletal, and lymphatic systems.

**Susceptibility** After the loss of maternal antibodies, susceptibility for rubella is general. Maternal transmission to the fetus is the greatest risk because the rubella virus can cause developmental defects. Natural infection and immunization generally confer lifelong immunity.

**Routes of Transmission**     Rubella virus is passed from person to person by direct contact with nasopharyngeal secretions or by inhalation of droplets from a sneeze or cough. Infants with **congenital rubella syndrome (CRS)** shed large amounts of the virus in their secretions so these secretions are highly contagious.

**Signs and Symptoms**     Typical symptoms include a rash on the face and neck that spreads to the limbs and trunk (Figure A-6). This rash is not easily seen on dark-skinned individuals. Infected persons also may experience a slight fever with a runny nose and sore throat, enlarged lymph nodes, and red eyes. Children typically have no serious side effects, although rubella in adults is considerably more serious. Younger females sometimes develop a self-limiting arthritis. More extreme side effects include **encephalitis, thrombocytopenia,** and **Guillain–Barré syndrome.** The most serious hazard is to the unborn child, who may suffer from heart defects, hearing impairment, and

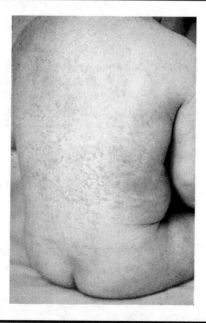

**FIGURE A-6** Rubella rash. (Photo courtesy of the Centers for Disease Control and Prevention.)

cataracts. Multiple defects are fairly common, and spontaneous abortion is possible.

**Patient Treatment**

Rubella is typically self-correcting, so treatment is rarely necessary. Care is primarily supportive, and is concentrated on controlling any fever and keeping the patient comfortable. When complications exist, they may need more aggressive treatment.

**Protective Measures**

When caring for a patient with rubella, standard and droplet precautions are indicated and effective hand washing is recommended.

**Immunizations**

The vaccine available for rubella is 98 to 99% effective and is combined with the mumps and measles vaccines (MMR). It is not recommended for pregnant females, and it is suggested that females who take the vaccine not become pregnant within 1 month after vaccination. The vaccine is not recommended for persons with a weakened immune system.

**Incubation Period**

The incubation period for rubella is 12 to 23 days, although symptoms typically appear within 16 to 18 days.

**Health Care Providers**

Health care providers should be screened for immunity and immunized as necessary. Females of child-bearing age should be immunized because of the risk of infecting an unborn baby. Standard and droplet precautions should be observed, and effective hand washing should take place.

# SALMONELLOSIS

**Causative Agent**

*Salmonella* is a bacterium that infects the gastrointestinal tract and the blood. Salmonellosis is a bacterial infection caused by one of the more than 2000 strands of *Salmonella*.

**Body Systems Affected**

Salmonellosis affects the gastrointestinal system and blood.

**Susceptibility**

Susceptibility for salmonellosis is general though children, the elderly, and those with a depressed immune system are at greater risk.

**Routes of Transmission**

Salmonellosis is typically considered a foodborne disease acquired through eating contaminated eggs, unpasteurized dairy products, or raw poultry. It may also be transmitted through contact with infected animals, especially turtles, iguanas, and other reptiles.

**Signs and Symptoms**   People who have salmonellosis report fever, chills, diarrhea, abdominal discomfort, and vomiting.

**Patient Treatment**   Care for salmonellosis is largely supportive. Fluids may be required to prevent dehydration.

**Protective Measures**   Standard precautions should be taken. Contact precautions should be taken if patient is incontinent. Effective hand washing is essential.

**Immunizations**   No vaccine for salmonellosis is available at this time.

**Incubation Period**   The expected incubation period for salmonellosis is 1 to 3 days.

**Health Care Providers**   Health care providers should be alert to the possibility of the disease, and should use standard precautions and practice good hand washing with all patients. Since reptiles, particularly iguanas have become popular pets, health care providers should be alert to the possibility of *Salmonella* infection.

## SCABIES

**Causative Agent**   The causative agent of scabies is *Sarcoptes scabiei*, a small **mite** that burrows into the skin. Scabies are grayish in color, nearly transparent and about the size of the period at the end of this sentence.

**Body Systems Affected**   Scabies affect the integumentary system. The mites typically begin by burrowing into the webs between fingers and toes, around the wrist, or navel. Later, the mites spread to other areas, including the groin, armpits, abdomen, and elbows.

**Susceptibility**   Susceptibility is general. Scabies does not discriminate with regard to age, race, or socioeconomic standing. Those who have been previously exposed may have fewer mites and their symptoms tend to develop faster (in 1 to 4 days versus 2 to 6 weeks for those who have never been exposed).

**Routes of Transmission**   Scabies is most frequently spread by direct skin-to-skin contact. It is possible to catch scabies indirectly through contaminated bedclothes and undergarments, but only if these items were contaminated by an infected person immediately prior to your touching them. Scabies may also be transmitted during sexual contact. It takes approximately 2 to 3 minutes for a mite to burrow into the skin.

**Signs and Symptoms**

The primary symptom of scabies is itching. People who become sensitive to the presence of scabies or their waste products may have large areas of reddened, inflamed, itching skin.

**Patient Treatment**

Care is largely supportive and includes replacing contaminated clothing. Skin lotions containing permethrin or crotamiton may be prescribed to control the itching.

**Protective Measures**

Standard precautions are indicated. Contact precautions should be taken for 24 hours after treatment and for environmental cleaning, which should include bagging all linens and contaminated clothing.

**Immunizations**

There is no vaccination for scabies at this time.

**Incubation Period**

Symptoms appear 2 to 6 weeks after exposure to scabies. An infected person will continue to spread scabies until all mites and eggs are destroyed.

**Health Care Providers**

Those who care for patients with scabies should take care to wear appropriate PPE, bag linens and contaminated clothing, and decontaminate all equipment that comes in contact with the patient.

# SEVERE ACUTE RESPIRATORY SYNDROME (SARS)

**Causative Agent**

The causative agent of SARS is a SARS-associated coronavirus (SARS-CoV).

**Body Systems Affected**

SARS, as its name would imply, primary affects the respiratory system.

**Susceptibility**

Those most susceptible to SARS are those who have been in close contact with an infected person.

**Routes of Transmission**

SARS is spread primarily through respiratory droplets and may be spread when a person touches an object contaminated with infected droplets, then touches the mucous membranes in the mouth, nose, or around the eyes.

**Signs and Symptoms**

Signs and symptoms of SARS include fever, body aches, headache, and respiratory symptoms, developing into pneumonia.

**Patient Treatment**

Antiviral medications are sometimes effective in treating SARS.

**Protective Measures**

Protective measures should include:

- Standard precautions, including thorough handwashing;
- Droplet precautions, including wearing gown and gloves for all contact;
- Airborne precautions, including using a NIOSH-approved N95 respirator; and
- Eye protection, worn anytime the caregiver is within 3 feet of the patient.

**Immunizations**

A vaccine for SARS is in the research phase.

**Incubation Period**

The incubation period for SARS is 2 to 7 days.

**Health Care Providers**

If a person who has recently traveled from a country in which SARS has been reported presents with flu-like symptoms, the local health department should be contacted. Early recognition, surveillance, and prevention activities significantly reduce the chances of an outbreak.

## SHIGELLOSIS

**Causative Agent**

Shigellosis is a bacterial infection that affects the lining of the intestinal tract, caused by infection with *Shigella* organisms.

**Body Systems Affected**

Shigellosis affects the gastrointestinal system and liver.

**Susceptibility**

Susceptibility for shigellosis is general, although more cases are reported in the summer months in areas with a cooler climate. The disease tends to be more common in children, ages 2 to 3 years.

**Routes of Transmission**

This disease is most commonly spread through direct contact with infected stool. Water and food may become contaminated, which allows an opportunity for waterborne and foodborne transmission.

|  |  |
|---|---|
| | When sexual practices allow contact with stool, opportunity also exists for sexual transmission. |
| Signs and Symptoms | Patients with shigellosis experience diarrhea, abdominal cramps, nausea and vomiting, painful bowel movements, fever, and loss of appetite. |
| Patient Treatment | Aggressive treatment for shigellosis is rarely indicated. IV fluids are sometimes needed to combat dehydration. Antibiotics may be helpful in severe cases. |
| Protective Measures | Standard precautions and thorough hand washing are indicated. Contact precautions should be taken if the patient is incontinent. |
| Immunizations | There is currently no vaccine for shigellosis. |
| Incubation Period | The incubation period for shigellosis ranges from 1 to 7 days, with the average being 2 to 3 days. |
| Health Care Providers | Health care providers should take standard precautions and observe contact precautions if the patient is incontinent. Hand washing is, as always, very important. |

## SYPHILIS

|  |  |
|---|---|
| Causative Agent | Syphilis is caused by the *Treponema pallidum* bacteria. An infection is caused first at the initially exposed site, then moves throughout the body, causing damage to multiple organs over time. |
| Body Systems Affected | Syphilis affects many organs, including the skin, eyes, and kidneys as well as the cardiovascular, skeletal, and central nervous systems. |
| Susceptibility | Susceptibility to syphilis is general. Approximately 30% of exposures result in infection. |
| Routes of Transmission | This disease is transmitted from the initial ulcer of an infected person to the skin or mucous membranes of the genital area, the mouth, or the anus of the sexual partner. It can also penetrate broken skin on other parts of the body. It may also be passed from a pregnant woman to her unborn child or transmitted via needlestick or blood transfusion. |

**Signs and Symptoms**

Syphilis presents in four stages (primary, secondary, latent, and tertiary). The first symptom of primary syphilis is the development of a **chancre** ulcer. This chancre usually develops 3 to 6 weeks after the initial exposure and is located on the part of the body initially exposed. If untreated, the disease may progress to the secondary stage.

Secondary syphilis is noted for its skin rash, which may occur on any part of the body, but nearly always includes the palms of the hands and soles of the feet. The rash presents as small red or brown lesions that contain active bacteria. Any contact with the broken skin of an infected person may spread the infection during this stage. Other symptoms include headache, fever, sore throat, fatigue, and swollen lymph nodes. Symptoms may continue sporadically for 1 to 2 years and may progress to latent syphilis if untreated.

Latent syphilis is a stage in which the syphilis is no longer contagious and no symptoms are present. Some patients relapse into secondary syphilis while others may progress to tertiary syphilis. There are usually no more relapses after 4 years.

The fourth stage, tertiary syphilis, can last for years or even decades. Complications include mental illness, blindness, central nervous system problems, heart disease, and even death. It is not contagious in this stage.

**Patient Treatment**

Antibiotics such as penicillin, erythromycin, and doxyclycline may be helpful. Other care is supportive.

**Protective Measures**

Standard precautions and thorough hand washing are essential. Caution should be used when handling soiled linens.

**Immunizations**

There is currently no vaccine for syphilis.

**Incubation Period**

Symptoms of syphilis may occur in as few as 10 days or as long as 3 months.

**Health Care Providers**

Health care providers should take care to avoid exposure to any body fluid, including the fluid from lesions. PPE and effective hand washing are essential.

## TETANUS

**Causative Agent**

Tetanus is an infection caused by *Clostridium tetani*, a bacteria found in almost anything lying on the ground, including the soil. *C. tetani* seems to thrive on rusty metal, so puncture wounds with rusty nails are a common cause of tetanus. *C. tetani* readily grows in wounds and produces a toxin that paralyzes muscles.

**Body Systems Affected**

Tetanus generally affects the musculoskeletal system by causing muscular stiffness and rigidity (Figure A-7).

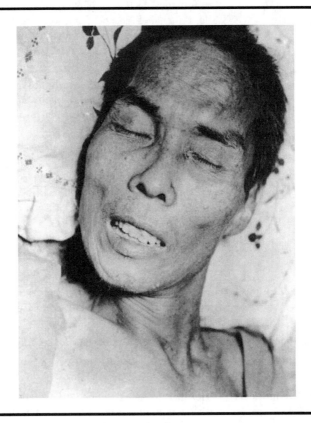

**FIGURE A-7** Tetanus. Note the muscular contraction of the jaw. (Photo courtesy of the Centers for Disease Control and Prevention.)

| | |
|---|---|
| **Susceptibility** | Susceptibility is general. |
| **Routes of Transmission** | Tetanus cannot be transmitted from person to person. It is generally transmitted through puncture wounds or cuts. |
| **Signs and Symptoms** | Symptoms of tetanus include fever, headache, difficulty in swallowing, and muscular stiffness in the neck and jaw-(thus the name lockjaw). |
| **Patient Treatment** | Care for patients experiencing symptoms of tetanus is mostly supportive. |
| **Protective Measures** | Since tetanus is not communicable from person to person, only standard precautions are necessary. |
| **Immunizations**  | Two agents are available. Tetanus immune globulin (TIG) is a concentrate of antibodies produced against tetanus toxin by immunized people. Another available agent is tetanus toxoid, which works by making the body produce antibodies to the toxin and protect one from future infections. Since immunity to tetanus wanes with time, periodic boosters are necessary. |
| **Incubation Period** | The incubation period for tetanus is typically 8 days, but may range from 3 days to 3 weeks. |
| **Health Care Providers** | Health care providers may have opportunity to counsel patients who may have been exposed to *C. tetani*. Patients who have received a small cut or puncture wound may defer treatment because of the perceived minor nature of the wound. Patients should be made aware of the danger of tetanus and of the importance of immunization. |

## TUBERCULOSIS

| | |
|---|---|
| **Causative Agent** | Tuberculosis is a bacterial disease caused by *Mycobacterium tuberculosis*. |
| **Body Systems Affected** | Tuberculosis can attack any part of the body. It usually affects the lungs, but it can also affect the renal, musculoskeletal, and lymphatic systems. |
| **Susceptibility** | Anyone can get tuberculosis, although immunocompromised persons and elderly persons are at greater risk. Those with diabetes or cancer may also be more susceptible. |

**Routes of Transmission**   Person-to-person transmission of tuberculosis is primarily through inhalation of droplets from a sneeze or cough. Persons may also become exposed to tuberculosis through prolonged, close exposure to an infected person. There are also a few recorded cases of exposure through direct infection through mucous membranes or broken skin, although this type exposure is uncommon.

**Signs and Symptoms**   Common symptoms include a persistent cough, fever, weight loss, fatigue, and night sweats. Some infected persons have no symptoms.

**Patient Treatment**   Initial care is primarily supportive. Recommended therapeutic care includes administration of a combination of medications that may include isoniazid, rifampin, ethambutol, pyrazinamide, and streptomycin.

**Protective Measures**   NIOSH-Approved HEPA respirators should be worn when in contact with patients who have active tuberculosis. Airborne and standard precautions are indicated.

**Immunizations**   There is currently no vaccine for tuberculosis. A skin test (**Mantoux test**) can show if TB bacteria are present.

**Incubation Period**   The incubation period for tuberculosis is typically between 4 and 12 weeks.

**Health Care Providers**   Health care providers, especially those in the prehospital or out-of-hospital setting, should be aware of the possibility of contracting TB from patients with an active cough. In situations in which a caregiver will be in a confined area with the patient for a prolonged period of time, caregivers should wear a HEPA mask.

---

# VANCOMYCIN–INTERMEDIATE/RESISTANT *STAPHYLOCOCCUS AUREUS* (VISA/VRSA)

**Causative Agent**   VRSA is caused by a bacteria, *Staphylococcus aureus*, that is resistant to many antibiotics. *Staph. aureus* is normally found on the skin and in the noses of healthy people. It occasionally causes infection, which may be minor or severe. Most staph bacteria are susceptible to vancomycin, but some have developed resistance, which means that vancomycin cannot harm them.

**Body Systems Affected**

A variety of body systems may be affected, depending on the location of the infection.

**Susceptibility**

VISA and VRSA are rare. Those who have multiple underlying health problems, prior MRSA, and/or recent exposure to vancomycin and other antimicrobial agents are at greater risk.

**Routes of Transmission**

VRSA is typically spread through direct contact with the hands of a health care provider or by environmental contamination.

**Signs and Symptoms**

Signs and symptoms are consistent with those of any infection.

**Patient Treatment**

VRSA and VISA may be treated with antibiotics other than vancomycin.

**Protective Measures**

Standard precautions, including wearing gloves, should be taken with all patients. Contact precautions should be observed when a patient is incontinent, and a gown should be worn when there is risk of soiling clothing. Most of all, thorough hand washing with soap and water or an alcohol-based rub is essential.

**Immunizations**

There is no vaccine for VRSA or VISA.

**Incubation Period**

The incubation period is unknown.

**Health Care Providers**

It is important that health care providers thoroughly wash their hands, observe standard and contact precautions, and actively work to reduce the number of hospital-associated infections.

## VANCOMYCIN-RESISTANT ENTEROCOCCI (VRE)

**Causative Agent**

Enterococci are part of the normal flora found in the intestinal tract. Whereas some species are relatively resistant to many commonly used antibiotic agents, most have been sensitive to vancomycin. When these species with resistance to other antibiotics become resistant to vancomycin, they have an advantage over other species in that they may replicate in the intestinal tract while others are eradicated.

| | |
|---|---|
| **Body Systems Affected** | A variety of body systems may be affected, depending on the location of the infection. |
| **Susceptibility** | Hospitalized patients, especially those in intensive-care units, are most susceptible to VRE. Specifically, those who have prolonged hospitalization, serious underlying medical conditions, urinary catheterization, or prior therapy with multiple antibiotics are at increased risk. |
| **Routes of Transmission** | VRE is typically spread through direct contact with the hands of a health care provider or by environmental contamination. |
| **Signs and Symptoms** | Signs and symptoms are consistent with those of any infection. |
| **Patient Treatment** | Treatment options for patients with VRE are limited, and are focused on preventing spread of the bacteria. |
| **Protective Measures** | Standard precautions, including wearing gloves, should be taken with all patients. Contact precautions should be observed when a patient is incontinent and a gown should be worn when there is risk of soiling clothing. Most of all, thorough hand washing with soap and water or an alcohol-based rub is essential. |
| **Immunizations** | There is no vaccine for VRE. |
| **Incubation Period** | The incubation period for VRE is unknown. |
| **Health Care Providers** | It is important that health care providers thoroughly wash their hands, observe standard and contact precautions, and actively work to reduce the number of hospital-associated infections. |

## BIBLIOGRAPHY

Centers for Disease Control and Prevention. (1989, June 23). Guidelines for prevention of transmission of human immunodeficiency virus and hepatis B virus to health-care and public safety workers. *Morbidity and Mortality Weekly Report, 38*(S-6).

Centers for Disease Control and Prevention. (1993, Aug. 6). Nosocomial enterococci resistant to vancomycin—United States, 1989–1993. *Morbidity and Mortality Weekly Report, 42*(30).

Centers for Disease Control and Prevention. (1999). MRSA—Methicillin resistant *Staphylococcus aureus* information for healthcare personnel. http://www.cdc.gov/ncidod/dhqp/ar_mrsa_healthcareFS.html.

Centers for Disease Control and Prevention. (1999, Dec. 31). Summary of notifiable diseases, United States, 1998. *Morbidity and Mortality Weekly Report, 47*(53).

Centers for Disease Control and Prevention. (2000, Feb. 4). Outbreaks of salmonella serotype enteritidis infection associated with eating raw or undercooked shell eggs–United States, 1996–1998. *Morbidity and Mortality Weekly Report, 49*(4).

Centers for Disease Control and Prevention. (2000, March 17). Hantavirus pulmonary syndrome—Panama, 1999–2000. *Morbidity and Mortality Weekly Report, 49*(10).

Centers for Disease Control and Prevention. (2000, April 14). Salmonellosis associated with chicks and ducklings—Michigan and Missouri, Spring, 1999. *Morbidity and Mortality Weekly Report, 49*(14).

Centers for Disease Control and Prevention. (2000, April 21). *Escherichia coli* O111:H8 outbreak among teenage campers—Texas, 1999. *Morbidity and Mortality Weekly Report, 49*(15).

Centers for Disease Control and Prevention. (2003). Vancomycin-intermediate/resistant *Staphylococcus aureus.* http://www.cdc.gov/ncidod/dhqp/ar_visavrsa.html.

Centers for Disease Control and Prevention. (2005). *Clostridium Difficile* general information. http://www.cdc.gov/ncidod/dhqp/id_CdiffFAQ_general.html.

Centers for Disease Control and Prevention. (2005). *Clostridium Difficile* information for healthcare providers. http://www.cdc.gov/ncidod/dhqp/id_Cdiff.html.

Centers for Disease Control and Prevention. (2005). Frequently asked questions about a new strain of *Clostridium difficile*. http://www.cdc.gov/ncidod/dhqp/id_CdiffFAQ_newstrain.html.

Centers for Disease Control and Prevention. (2005, April 4). Frequently asked questions about plague. Atlanta: Author.

Centers for Disease Control and Prevention. (2005, May 3). Fact sheet: Basic information about SARS. http://www.cdc.gov/ncidod/sars/factsheet.htm.

Centers for Disease Control and Prevention. (2005, Oct. 6). Diarrheagenic *Escherichia coli*. http://www.cdc.gov/ncidod/dbmd/diseaseinfo/diarrecoli_t.htm.

Centers for Disease Control and Prevention. (2005, Oct. 25). Enterotoxigenic *Escherichia coli* (ETEC). http://www.cdc.gov/ncidod/dbmd/diseaseinfo/etec_g.htm.

Centers for Disease Control and Prevention. (2005). What is CDC doing about MRSA? http://www.cdc.gov/ncidod/dbmd/diseaseinfo/ etec_g.htm.

Centers for Disease Control and Prevention. Web site. http://www.cdc.gov.

Cockrum, E. L. (1997). *Rabies, lyme disease, Hantavirus and other animal-borne human diseases in the United States and Canada.* Tucson, AZ: Fisher Books.

The Corporation of the County of Oxford, Ontario, Canada. (2000). *Clostridium difficile.* http://www.county.oxford.on.ca/healthservices/ ocbh/cidc/clostridium.asp.

Damjanov, I. (2000). *Pathology for the health-related professions.* Philadelphia: Saunders.

Epimmune. Web site. http://www.epimmune.com.

Falk, Pamela S. (2000, July). How can VRE Infections be prevented in surgery? *Infection Control Today.* http://www.infectioncontroltoday. com/articles/071feat3.html.

The Hepatitis Information Network. Web site. http://www.hepnet.com.

Infection Control Today. (2005, Nov. 3). With or without pandemic scenario, flu is a serious health threat. *Infection Control Today.* http://www. infectioncontroltoday.com/hotnews/5bh38321560376.html.

Kennamer, M. A. (2005, Winter). Bird flu: What's all the fuss about? *What's Happening in EMS Online Newsletter.* Clifton Park, NY: Thomson Delmar Learning. http://emarketing.delmarlearning.com/ems/EMS_ news_dec05_feature.asp.

Levy, D. (2004, Jan. 16). Medical encyclopedia: *E. coli* enteritis. *Medline Plus.* http://www.nlm.nih.gov/medlineplus/ency/article/000296.htm.

Kids Health. Web site. http://www.kidshealth.org.

Manitoba Public Health Communicable Disease Control Unit. (2001, November). Vancomycin resistant enterococci (VRE).

Mayo Clinic. (2004, Oct. 4). SARS. http://www.mayoclinic.com/health/sars/ DS00501.

National Fire Academy, (1992). *Infection control for emergency response personnel: The supervisor's role.* Emmitsburg, MD: Author.

Neighbors, M., & Tannehill-Jones, R. (2006). *Human diseases* (2nd ed.). Clifton Park, NY: Thomson Delmar Learning.

New York State Department of Health. (2004). Methicillin resistant *Staphylococcus aureus* (MRSA). http://www.health.state.ny.us/ nysdoh/communicable_diseases/en/mrsa.htm.

Public Health Agency of Canada. (2001). Material Safety Data Sheet—
    Infectious Substances. http://phac-aspc.gc.ca/msds-ftss/msds36e.html.

New York State Department of Health. Web site. http://www.health.state.ny.us.

NZ Dermnet. Web site. http://www.dermnet.org.nz.

Smith, P. W. (1994). *Infection control in long-term care facilities.* (2nd ed.).
    Clifton Park, NY: Thomson Delmar Learning.

South Dakota Department of Health. Web site. http://www.state.sd.us/doh.

Sugar, A. M., & Lyman, C. A. (1997). *A practical guide to medically important
    fungi and the diseases they cause.* Philadelphia: Lippincott-Raven.

Thibodeau, G. A., & Patton, K. T. (1999). *Anatomy and physiology.* (4th ed.).
    St. Louis: Mosby.

Web MD Health. Web site. http://www.webmd.com.

World Health Organization. Web site. http://www.who.int.

# Answers to Questions for Discussion

The answers provided are intended to stimulate further discussion and are not intended as a definitive answer to the questions presented. The answers should, however, assist the reader in understanding the concepts presented.

## CHAPTER 1

1. What diseases have increased public awareness of infection control over the past few years?

   *Several diseases have been highlighted in the media, including SARS, avian flu, anthrax, and others.*

2. What simple infection control procedure helped Dr. Ignaz Semmelweis save a number of lives in the 1800s?

   *The simple procedure of hand washing helped Dr. Semmelweis reduce the death rate due to infection at his hospital.*

3. List three pioneers in the field of infection control.

   *Ignaz Semmelweis proved that hand washing could prevent the spread of infection. Louis Pasteur's background in physics and chemistry led him to discover some of the basic principles of microbiology as we know it today. Joseph Lister applied Pasteur's principles and initiated the use of antiseptics.*

4. List at least three diseases that should concern health care workers today.

   *Many diseases should be of concern. Hepatitis C is certainly a threat to health care providers and should warrant concern. Other diseases such as hepatitis B, hepatitis non-ABC, HIV, and others should be of concern as well.*

## CHAPTER 2

1. List three things required by OSHA regarding infection control.

   *OSHA mandates each employer with category I employees to develop an exposure control plan and offer hepatitis B vaccinations at no charge to the employee. Standards on personal protective equipment (PPE), record-keeping, training, and work practices were also developed by OSHA.*

2. What is the intent of the Ryan White CARE Act?

   *The Ryan White Comprehensive AIDS Resources Emergency Act of 1990 gives employees the right to learn if they were exposed to infectious disease while caring for a patient.*

3. Differentiate between states covered under state plans and states covered under federal OSHA jurisdiction.

   *State plan states must have a plan that meets or exceeds federal OSHA standards.*

4. List four components of a successful negligence lawsuit.
   - *Duty to act*
   - *Breach of duty*
   - *Damages*
   - *Proximate cause*

5. Describe the intent of the Americans with Disabilities Act (ADA).

   *The ADA is intended to protect individuals with disabilities from discrimination in hiring and advancement, job training, and employee compensation. It also provides equal access to public accommodations and commercial facilities.*

6. Explain why it is important to meet standards recognized by leading agencies in the infection control field.

   *Although the standards from these agencies may not carry the weight of law, an injured party may bring a civil suit on the grounds that expected standards were not met.*

# CHAPTER 3

1. Are all infectious diseases communicable? Explain your answer.

   *No. Some infectious diseases may not be considered person-to-person transmissible. For example, hantavirus is an infectious disease, but it cannot be transmitted person to person.*

2. Is a person more likely to become infected with HIV through direct or indirect contact? Explain your answer.

   *Since HIV is so weak outside the confines of the human body, indirect contact is highly unlikely.*

3. If you are exposed to a person with HIV today and have a negative blood test tomorrow, are you considered "safe"?

   *No. It may take weeks or months for a person to seroconvert and show a positive blood test. One negative test does not clear the person from infection.*

4. Name at least three ways diseases may be transmitted.

*Diseases may be transmitted person to person through airborne, bloodborne, vector borne, or sexual transmission.*

5. List at least four causes of infectious disease.

*Infectious disease may be caused by bacteria, viruses, fungi, rickettsia, or helminths.*

## CHAPTER 4

1. List and describe some of the key anatomical structures of the immune system.

*The immune system is comprised of organs and structures from several organ systems, including the integumentary, respiratory, gastrointestinal, and lymphatic systems. The tonsils protect the entrance of the respiratory system from invading pathogens. Lymph nodes filter harmful substances, and lymphatic vessels transport lymphatic fluid. The thymus produces T lymphocytes, and the spleen serves as the site of development for monocytes and lymphocytes. The appendix is thought to help prevent disease by harboring nonpathogenic bacteria, and the skin serves as a barrier that protects the body from invasion by external pathogens.*

2. Describe the process of phagocytosis and explain why it results in the production of pus.

*Phagocytes attack and ingest invading pathogens by trapping them with arm-like projections and forming a sac around them. Once in the sac, pathogens are chemically destroyed. Phagocytes have a short life span. Once their job is done, phagocytes die and aggregate as pus, which is readily absorbed into the surrounding tissues.*

3. Which lasts longer, passive or active immunity? Why?

*Active immunity lasts longer than passive immunity. Since the immunity is active, it means the body can produce antibodies to a certain antigen. This ability to produce antibodies makes active immunity longer acting than passive immunity, which is more immediate, but shorter acting.*

4. Of antigens and antibodies, which are more specific? Why?

*Antibodies are more specific. Antigens mark cells as self or nonself. Antibodies are specific to only one antigen.*

5. List several signs and symptoms of infections. Discuss why these signs appear.

*Characteristic signs of infection include hot, swollen, and reddened skin. These signs are caused by increased blood flow and vascular permeability in the affected area.*

## CHAPTER 5

1. List at least four examples of common engineering controls.

   *Examples of engineering controls include the placement of sharps containers, eye wash stations, handwashing facilities, and storage of hazardous chemicals.*

2. List at least four examples of safe work practices.

   *Safe work practices include hand washing, using personal protective equipment, not applying lip balm, and not smoking or eating in a work area.*

3. Who is responsible for ensuring that safe work practices are enforced?

   *Although each employee should be responsible for safe work practices, enforcement is the responsibility of the employer.*

4. Describe the differences in standard precautions and transmission-based precautions.

   *Standard precautions are used with all patients and advocate isolation from all body fluids (except sweat), nonintact skin, and mucous membranes. Transmission-based precautions are used for patients with a highly transmissible pathogen and may include airborne, droplet, and contact precautions.*

5. List and describe the three major types of transmission-based precautions.

   *Airborne precautions are used with patients who are known or suspected to be infected with an airborne infectious disease. Emphasis is on respiratory protection and patient placement. Droplet precautions are used to protect from inhaling large particle droplets of moisture that carry contaminants. Isolation and respiratory protection are indicated. Contact precautions are used to protect against infection caused by coming in contact with an infected person or his or her personal items. Isolation from other patients is preferred, and appropriate BSI is indicated.*

6. Explain why body substance isolation (BSI) is generally the preferred method of isolation used by prehospital and out-of-hospital providers.

   *BSI contends that any body substance is potentially infectious and health care providers should isolate themselves from any potentially infectious substance. In areas where there is little control over the environment in which patient care takes place, this maximal protection helps protect health care providers from unexpected exposures.*

7. Who is responsible for laundering or disposing of uniforms contaminated with blood or other potentially infectious materials?

*The responsibility for laundering or replacing uniforms is that of the employer.*

8. List and describe the three components of the personal health system.

*A comprehensive system of personal health should include pre-entry physical examinations, vaccinations, and return-to-work authorizations.*

9. List the contraindications of the hepatitis B vaccine.

*The hepatitis B vaccine should not be taken by those who are pregnant, nursing an infant, or sensitive to yeast or any of its components.*

10. Explain the procedure for cleaning up spilled blood.

*Once appropriate personal protective equipment is donned, care should be taken to contain the spill. One way to achieve this is to cover the spill with paper towels. Once contained, the spill may be absorbed with additional paper towels and placed in a biohazard bag for disposal. A mixture of common household bleach (sodium hypochlorite) and water should be used to further disinfect the affected area. The recommended mixture of bleach to water is between 1:10 and 1:100.*

11. Describe the three categories set forth by the Spaulding Classification System.

- *Critical—These are items that penetrate tissue. They must be sterilized.*
- *Semicritical—This is for items that contact, but do not penetrate, mucous membranes or nonintact skin. They require a high-level disinfection.*
- *Noncritical—These are items that contact intact skin, requiring only cleaning and intermediate-level disinfection.*

12. *Differentiate between cleaning, disinfecting, and sterilizing.*

*Cleaning involves removing debris and reducing the number of microorganisms present. Disinfecting is the act of applying a chemical disinfectant, either by spraying or immersion, to the surface of an object. Sterilization is the process of making an object free from all live microorganisms, usually with the use of gas or steam.*

## CHAPTER 6

1. Describe at least three cases in which biological weapons were used in warfare.

- *British used smallpox during the French and Indian War.*
- *Germans spread glanders during WWI.*
- *Japanese dropped plague-infested fleas on China during WWII.*

2. Compare and contrast bioterrorism and biological warfare in terms of delivery systems, agents, and motive.

|  | Bioterrorism | Biological Warfare |
|---|---|---|
| Sponsorship | Anyone | State-sponsored |
| Quantity | Small quantity | Large quantity |
| Delivery | Multiple methods, with varying precision | Bombs, missiles, or spray systems, with great precision |
| Motivation | Make a statement or undermine authority | Win a war |

3. Why have biological weapons not been used widely in warfare?

Biological weapons have some distinct disadvantages, including that they are impossible to control once released and may backfire on the ones releasing them. Conditions must also be right for successful use.

4. What are two advantages to biological warfare?

They do not destroy buildings or infrastructure, and they are relatively cheap compared with conventional weapons.

5. Differentiate between Category A, B, and C agents; name at least two examples of each.

| Category | Description | Examples |
|---|---|---|
| Category A | • Easily transmitted person to person<br>• May result in high mortality rates or have major public health impact.<br>• Require special action for public preparedness. | • Anthrax<br>• Botulism<br>• Plague<br>• Smallpox<br>• Tularemia<br>• Viral hemorrhagic fevers |
| Category B | • Moderately easy to disseminate.<br>• Result in moderate morbidity and low mortality rates.<br>• Require special enhancements to the CDC's capacity | • Brucellosis<br>• Glanders<br>• Psittacosis |
| Category C | • Emerging pathogens that may be engineered for future mass dissemination | • Nipah virus<br>• Hantavirus |

6. List the six category A agents.
   - *Anthrax*
   - *Botulism*
   - *Plague*
   - *Smallpox*
   - *Tularemia*
   - *Viral hemorrhagic fevers*

7. Describe how to make an agent a respirable aerosol.
   *This requires four components:*
   - *Agent—process so that it may be aerosolized.*
   - *Delivery system—device in which agent is carried.*
   - *Dissemination device—something with which to distribute the aerosolized agent.*
   - *Weather or microclimate—cloud cover, lack of rain, etc.*

8. Faced with a bioterrorism incident, what is your greatest priority?
   *A health care provider's greatest priority should always be personal safety.*

9. How can you best protect yourself against foodborne pathogens?
   *The best defense against foodborne pathogens is thoroughly cooking food.*

10. How can you best protect yourself from waterborne pathogens?
    *Waterborne pathogens can usually be killed by boiling.*

## CHAPTER 7

1. Why is it harder to determine exposure to airborne transmitted diseases than exposure to bloodborne transmitted diseases?
   *The method of travel for bloodborne diseases is more apparent and easier to determine than that of airborne transmitted diseases. In essence, blood is easier to see than airborne droplets in a sneeze or cough.*

2. What two things are necessary to determine that an exposure occurred?
   *A method of travel and a portal of entry should be determined to indicate exposure.*

3. Why would someone who rides in an ambulance carrying a patient with an airborne communicable disease be considered to have been exposed? Would someone who rides in a car with that same person be considered exposed? Why or why not?
   *Persons who occupy a small space with someone with an airborne transmissible disease are, because of the close quarters, considered*

*to have been exposed. This holds true both in an ambulance and in a car.*

## CHAPTER 8

1. How long must exposure records be kept by the employer?

   *Exposure records must be kept for the length of employment plus 30 years.*

2. What is the first priority after an exposure?

   *The first priority after an exposure should be immediate first aid treatment, including cleansing wounds and controlling bleeding.*

3. Can an employer fire an employee for contracting a communicable disease while off duty?

   *To fire an employee for contracting a communicable disease would violate the provisions of the Americans with Disabilities Act, which lists infectious disease as a disability. Job duties may be adjusted or medical leave may be granted depending on the situation and requirements of the job.*

4. List at least five signs or symptoms of stress.

   *Common signs and symptoms of stress include irritability, fatigue, lack of concentration, insomnia, and depression.*

5. Discuss several strategies for stress reduction.

   *People choose to cope with stress in different ways. Health care providers may choose to use a combination of counseling, education, and physical strategies to help reduce stress levels.*

# Glossary

**acquired immunity**—type of specific immunity that one is not born with. May be artificial (caused by immunization) or natural (resulting from nondeliberate exposure to antigens after birth).

**acquired immunodeficiency syndrome (AIDS)**—fatal illness caused by infection with the human immunodeficiency virus (HIV).

**active immunity**—refers to an individual who has the ability to produce antibodies to a certain antigen.

**adsorb**—to attract and retain another material.

**airborne precautions**—isolation method for patients known or suspected to be infected with airborne transmissible diseases; emphasis is placed on patient placement and respiratory protection.

**airborne transmission**—refers to the transmission of microorganisms by a cough or sneeze.

**American Institute of Architects (AIA)**—organization that represents the professional interests of American architects.

**Americans with Disabilities Act (ADA)**—legislation designed to prohibit discrimination against persons with disabilities. "Contagious disease" is specifically listed as a qualifying disability.

**antibodies**—proteins that attach themselves to antigens to mark them for destruction.

**antigens**—chemical markers that identify cells as self (human) or nonself (foreign).

**Association for Professionals in Infection Control and Epidemiology (APIC)**—association dedicated to excellence in the prevention and control of infections and related adverse outcomes.

**antiviral**—pertains to something that opposes, interferes with replication of, or weakens the action of a virus.

**aphasia**—loss of the ability to speak.

**asymptomatic**—without symptoms.

**attenuated**—thinned, reduced, or weakened.

**autoimmune response**—cells or antibodies created by and working against the body's own tissues.

194

**bacteria**—a type of living microorganism that can produce disease in a host. Bacteria can self-produce, and some produce toxins that are harmful to their host.

**B lymphocytes**—white blood cells primarily responsible for humoral immunity.

**basophils**—phagocytic leukocytes similar in form and function to mast cells.

**Bell's palsy**—unilateral paralysis of facial muscles caused by dysfunction of the seventh cranial nerve.

**biohazard container**—a puncture-resistant container used for the proper disposal of contaminated needles and other contaminated items.

**biological terrorism**—intentional or threatened use of biological agents to make a statement or to undermine authority. *See also* bioterrorism.

**biological warfare**—intentional use of bacteria, viruses, or toxins to cause death or disease in humans, plants, or animals. It is usually state-sponsored and delivered in large quantities.

**bioterrorism**—intentional or threatened use of biological agents to make a statement or to undermine authority. *See also* biological terrorism.

**bloodborne transmission**—pertains to the spread of microorganisms present in human blood that are capable of causing disease.

**body substance isolation (BSI)**—the school of thought regarding personal protective equipment regards any substance related to the body as infectious, and advocates placing a barrier between the employee and the substance.

**breach of duty**—failure to meet the obligation of providing care.

**cancerous**—pertaining to a malignant neoplasm.

**casual contact**—everyday contact with those who live, work, or go to school together. *See also* household contact.

**Category A agent**—an organism that risks national security because of its ability to be transmitted from person to person. It may result in high mortality rates or have a major public health impact, may cause public panic, and may require special action for public health preparedness. Agents include anthrax, botulism, plague, smallpox, tularemia, and viral hemorrhagic fevers.

**Category B agent**—a second-priority agent that is moderately easy to disseminate, results in moderate morbidity and low mortality rates, and requires special enhancements to the CDC's capacity. Agents in this category include brucellosis, food and water safety threats, glanders, psittacosis, and ricin.

**Category C agent**—a third-priority agent that includes emerging pathogens that may be engineered for future mass dissemination based on availability, ease of production, and potential for major health impact and high morbidity and mortality rates. Specific agents include such pathogens as Nipah virus and hantavirus.

**category 1 employee**—an OSHA term that refers to an employee who is considered at the greatest risk of occupational exposure to communicable disease.

**causative agent**—an agent that causes a particular disease.

**cell-mediated immunity**—immunity provided by T cells.

**Centers for Disease Control and Prevention (CDC)**—division of the U.S. Department of Health and Human Services that conducts ongoing research on infection control issues.

**chancre**—the primary sore or lesion of syphillis.

**chemotaxis**—movement in response to chemical stimulation.

**chronic infection**—an invasion by a microorganism, causing contamination, that is expected to last for a long time.

**civil liability**—a wrong against another individual for which remedy damages are awarded. Typically in infection control issues the liability is a result of not meeting an established standard.

**cleaning**—involves removing debris and reducing the number of microorganisms present.

**communicable disease**—an infectious disease that can be transmitted from one person to another.

**communicable period**—period after an infection when an infectious agent can be transmitted to another host.

**complement proteins**—group of approximately 20 inactivated plasma proteins, called *complement*, which circulate in the blood. When activated, complement proteins cause rupture of the cell that triggered it.

**congenital rubella syndrome (CRS)**—high incidence of congenital birth defects resulting from maternal infection with rubella during the first trimester.

**conjunctivitis**—inflammation of the membrane lining of the eyelids, and covering the eyeball.

**contact precautions**—CDC guidelines for limiting contact with an infected person or his/her personal items.

**critical**—classification in the Spaulding Classification System used for items that penetrate tissue and must be sterilized.

**cross-contamination**—refers to contamination between patients or between a health care provider and a patient.

**damages**—monetary or other loss.

**delivery system**—a vehicle in which a dissemination device is transported.

**Department of Homeland Security (DHS)**—Federal agency designed to help prevent, protect against, and respond to acts of terrorism on U.S. soil.

**debridement**—removal of dead tissue or foreign matter from a wound.

**designated officer**—required by the Ryan White CARE Act of 1990. This person is a liaison between the employee and the physician or hospital when an exposure takes place.

**direct transmission**—transmission of a disease from one person to another through direct contact with infected blood, body fluids, or other infectious material.

**disease period**—time between onset of symptoms and resolution of symptoms.

**disinfection**—applying a chemical disinfectant to the surface by spraying or immersion.

**disseminated intravascular coagulation (DIC)**—hemorrhagic syndrome that occurs following an uncontrolled activation of clotting factors.

**dissemination device**—mechanism to deliver a respirable aerosol.

**dormant**—inactive.

**droplet precautions**—CDC guidelines intended to protect the health care provider from inhaling large particle droplets of moisture carrying contaminants.

**duty to act**—refers to the duty of a caregiver to provide appropriate medical care.

**dysuria**—difficulty with or pain on urination.

**encephalitis**—inflammation of the brain.

**endogenous flora**—microbial flora normally existing in the body of the host.

**engineering controls**—actions taken by the employer to make the workplace safer by engineering safety directly into the workplace.

**enteric**—referring to the intestine.

**enterohemorrhagic**—refers to bleeding within or from the intestines.

**environmentally resistant**—durable or able to survive outside the confines of the human body.

**epididymitis**—inflammation of the epididymis.

**essential functions**—actions or attributes the employee must meet, with or without accommodation, to fulfill the duties of a job.

**exogenous flora**—microbial flora normally existing outside the body of the host.

**exposure**—contact with blood, body fluids, or potentially infectious material.

**exposure control plan**—written document required by OSHA that outlines the employer's infection control plan.

**exposure report form**—standard form used by an employee to report an occupational exposure.

**exudates**—fluid that seeps out of a tissue or its capillaries, usually because of injury or inflammation.

**first aid**—general measures taken in the minutes after an accident or illness that might include actions such as controlling bleeding and cleaning wounds.

**fit-tested**—procedure required to ensure the proper fit of a particulate respirator.

**foodborne**—pathogen spread through food.

**fungus**—plant-like organism that may grow as single cells (e.g., yeast) or as multicellular colonies (e.g., mold).

**Guillain-Barré syndrome**—acute, progressive disease that affects the spinal nerves.

**health care-associated infection (HAI)**—infection acquired in a health care facility. *Also called* nosocomial infection.

**helminths**—parasitic worms.

**helper T cells**—specialized T cells that have a receptor for immunoglobulin M antibodies.

**hemolytic-uremic syndrome**—hemolytic anemia and thrombocytopenia occurring with acute renal failure. Associated with infection, complications of pregnancy following normal delivery, or oral contraceptive use.

**hepatitis B virus (HBV)**—a bloodborne virus that poses a serious threat to employees at risk for occupational exposure. The hepatitis B virus is very dangerous because it can stay active outside the body for long periods of time.

**hepatitis C virus (HCV)**—virus that affects the liver. Currently the most common chronic bloodborne infection in the United States.

**household contact**—everyday contact with those who live, work, or go to school together. *See also* casual contact.

**humoral immunity**—type of specific immunity that occurs within plasma. *Also called* antibody-mediated immunity.

**hygiene**—practices that promote cleanliness and good health.

**incubation period**—the time from the exposure to a disease until the first appearance of symptoms.

**indirect transmission**—transmission of a disease from one person to another without direct contact.

**infectious disease**—a disease that results from an invasion of a host from a disease-producing organism. This organism may be in the form of a virus, bacteria, fungus, or parasite.

**inflammatory response**—second line of protection against pathogens. The inflammatory response uses specialized leukocytes, called neutrophils and macrophages, to find and destroy invading pathogens through a process called phagocytosis.

**inherited immunity**—specific immunity that is acquired in utero.

**integumentary system**—the skin and its structures.

**interferon**—a protein that defends against viral infections. By inhibiting the ability of a virus to cause a disease, interferon prevents viruses from replicating in cells.

**Joint Commission on Accreditation of Healthcare Organizations (JCAHO)**—national organization responsible for the accreditation of health care facilities.

**killer T cells**—lymphocytes able to recognize, bind to, and kill antigens located on the surface of pathogenic cells. By releasing lymphotoxin, a powerful poison, killer T cells eliminate pathogens directly.

**Koplik's spots**—distinctive, small, irregular, red spots with a bluish or white speck in the center. Found on the buccal and lingual mucosa during early stages of measles. Often a telltale sign of measles.

**lacrimation**—secretion of tears.

**latent period**—period after infection when an infectious agent cannot be transmitted to another host.

**lesion**—pathologic change in the tissues, which may be benign or malignant.

**leukocytes**—white blood cells whose function is to protect the body against pathogens.

**lymphocytes**—types of leukocyte formed in bone marrow. Lymphocytes participate in immunity.

**lymphotoxins**—toxins from T lymphocytes that damage many cell types.

**lysozyme**—enzyme destructive to cell walls of certain bacteria.

**macrophage**—type of phagocyte that migrates out of the bloodstream and grows to several times its original size. Found in the alveoli, lymph nodes, brain, liver, and spleen, macrophages ingest invading and dead cells.

**Mantoux test**—diagnostic test for tuberculosis that involves the intradermal injection of tuberculin bacteria particles.

**mast cells**—found in all tissues of the body, mast cells play a role in the inflammatory process.

**method of travel**—the means through which pathogens enter the body.

**microclimate**—refers to conditions within an area such as a building.

**mite**—transparent or semitransparent arthropod, which may be parasitic on humans or animals, causing skin irritations.

**mitotic**—relating to the process of reproduction of cells caused by indirect cell division.

**mode of transmission**—the means through which pathogens enter the body. *See also* method of travel.

**mutate**—the act of the DNA structure being changed, resulting in a new character trait not found in the parental type.

**myalgia**—muscle pain.

**myoclonus**—referring to one or a series of shock-like contractions of a muscle group, caused by a central nervous system lesion.

**National Institute for Occupational Safety and Health (NIOSH)**—the federal agency responsible for conducting research and making recommendations for the prevention of work-related injury and illness. NIOSH is part of the Centers for Disease Control and Prevention (CDC) in the Department of Health and Human Services.

**natural killer cells**—type of lymphocyte that recognizes and destroys infected or tumor cells. Natural killer cells do not have to be activated by an external antigen, so they are considered nonspecific.

**necrosis**—pertaining to cell death.

**negligence**—act of being neglectful, or not acting as a health care provider of similar experience and training would.

**neutrophils**—the most numerous of the phagocytes, neutrophils are mature white blood cells that ingest the microorganisms through phagocytosis and die within 1 or 2 days.

**NIOSH-approved respirator**—a particulate respirator approved by the National Institute for Occupational Safety and Health.

**noncritical**—classification in the Spaulding Classification System used for items that contact intact skin, requiring only cleaning and intermediate-level disinfection.

**nonsteroidal antiinflammatory drugs (NSAIDs)**—group of over-the-counter medications commonly used to reduce swelling.

**nosocomial infections**—infection originating in a hospital.

**notification by request**—made by any employee who is potentially exposed to a communicable disease while providing patient care.

**nuchal rigidity**—stiffness of the neck.

**nymph**—developmental stage in certain arthropods, resembling an adult.

**occupational exposure**—exposure of an employee to communicable disease while performing job-related duties.

**Occupational Safety and Health Administration (OSHA)**—an organization charged with the protection of employees in the workplace.

**oocyst**—dormant form of cryptosporidium; a parasitic protozoan that lives in the intestines of people and animals.

**other potentially infectious material (OPIM)** — material, other than blood, that may reasonably be expected to be infectious.

**other than serious violation** — an OSHA violation that has a direct relationship to safety and health, but is not likely to cause death or serious injury. A proposed penalty of up to $7000 may be levied.

**pandemic** — epidemic over a wide area or affecting a large population.

**parasitic** — referring to organisms that live in or on the body of the host, and gain some advantage from the host.

**paresthesia** — abnormal sensation (burning, prickling, etc.) for no apparent reason.

**particulate respirator** — NIOSH-approved device that may be used to protect one from airborne hazards.

**passive immunity** — refers to immunity from an outside source or transferred to someone who was not previously immune. Passive immunity provides temporary, but immediate, protection.

**pathogenic** — causing disease or abnormality.

**pediculicide** — agent used to destroy lice.

**pelvic inflammatory disease (PID)** — inflammation of some or all of the pelvic reproductive organs.

**peripheral neuropathy** — disorder affecting the peripheral or autonomic nervous system.

**personal health** — a three-part plan consisting of physical examinations, vaccinations, and authorization to return to duty or work.

**personal protective equipment (PPE)** — any equipment used to protect the employee from occupational exposure to blood and body fluid.

**petechial rash** — rash marked by small hemorrhages within the skin.

**phagocytosis** — inflammatory process in which phagocytes (cells capable of phagocytosis) attack and ingest the invading agent.

**photophobia** — abnormal intolerance to light.

**portal of entry** — path through which pathogens gain entry into the body.

**postexposure testing and follow-up** — a series of laboratory tests and medical exams that are performed after an exposure incident.

**pre-entry physical exam** — exam frequently required before entry into service.

**prodromal** — early symptom of a disease.

**prophylaxis** — preventive treatment.

**prostatitis** — inflammation of the prostate.

**protozoans** — the simplest organisms in the animal kingdom. Many are single-celled, although some colonize.

**proximate cause** — relation between an inappropriate action or inaction and damages. To prove negligence one must show that a breach of duty caused damages.

**public health system**—organizations and entities that contribute to the public health of communities.

**purulent**—containing or consisting of pus.

**qualified individual with a disability**—a person who meets the requisite skill, education, experience, and other job-related requirements of the position the individual holds or desires and who, with or without reasonable accommodations, can perform the essential functions of the job.

**reasonable accommodation**—a modification to the work environment that enables a person with a disability to perform the essential functions of a job.

**repeat violation**—a violation of any OSHA standard, rule, or order for which, on reinspection, the same or a similar violation is found. Repeat violations may result in penalties of up to $70,000.

**replicate**—to duplicate or reproduce.

**respirable aerosol**—a gaseous suspension of fine solid or liquid particles that is capable of being inhaled.

**return-to-work authorization**—medical approval to return to work/duty after an exposure incident or any illness requiring the employee to miss work for medical reasons.

**rickettsia**—parasitical bacteria that depend on living cells for growth.

**routine notification**—provided by the treating facility or hospital to employees who are exposed to a patient found to have an airborne communicable disease.

**Ryan White Comprehensive Aids Resources Emergency (CARE) Act of 1990**—landmark legislation that gives certain employees the right to learn if they were exposed to infectious disease in the course of caring for a patient.

**safe work practices**—rules of conduct, set forth by an employer's standard operating procedure or employee handbook, governing practices and procedures that make the workplace safer.

**saprophytic**—referring to an organism that grows on dead organic matter.

**sebum**—oily substance secreted by the sebaceous glands.

**semicritical**—classification in the Spaulding Classification System used for items that contact, but do not penetrate, mucous membranes or nonintact skin. These items require a high level of disinfection.

**septic arthritis**—acute inflammation of synovial membranes caused by bacterial infection.

**serious violation**—an OSHA violation for which there is substantial probability that death or physical harm could result, and that the employer knew, or should have known, that the hazard existed. The penalty is $7000 per occurrence.

**seroconversion**—a change in the status of a person's serum test.

**sexual transmission**—the passing of a disease through any type of sexual contact.

**sexually transmitted disease (STD)**—disease transmitted through sexual contact.

**sharps container**—puncture-resistant and leak-proof biohazard container intended for discarded needles, scalpels, and other sharps.

**Spaulding Classification System**—system developed by Dr. Earl Spaulding intended to determine appropriate methods for preparing supplies and instruments for patient use based on the item's intended use. Classifications include critical, semicritical, and noncritical.

**specific immunity**—immunity against specific foreign pathogens.

**spores**—a dormant nonproductive form of a pathogen.

**standard of care**—level of care expected of a given level of health care provider. A basis for comparison.

**Standard Precautions**—CDC recommendations that apply to all patients receiving care in hospitals. These precautions apply to contact with blood, all body fluids (with the exception of sweat), nonintact skin, and mucous membranes.

**sterilization**—process of making an object free from all microorganisms, usually with the use of gas or steam.

**susceptible**—at risk of infection.

**systemic bacteremia**—presence of bacteria in circulating blood.

**T lymphocytes**—specialized lymphocytes that develop in the thymus, and typically reside in the spleen and lymph nodes; responsible for cell-mediated immunity.

**T suppressor cells**—specialized lymphocytes that regulate the function of B cells and other T cells.

**therapeutic**—related to curing or treating a disease or condition.

**thrombocytopenia**—condition of having an abnormally small number of platelets in the circulating blood.

**transmission-based precautions**—CDC recommendations used with patients known or suspected to be infected with highly transmissible or epidemiologically important pathogens. One or more of three types of transmission-based precautions may be used, depending on the way a given disease is transmitted.

**tuberculosis (TB)**—a lower respiratory tract infection that is spread through airborne water droplets.

**tumor**—a new growth of tissue in which cell multiplication is uncontrolled.

**undue hardship**—an accommodation requiring significant expense or difficulty to an employer, for which the employer may legally refuse to provide under the terms of the ADA.

**universal biohazard symbol**—symbol that conforms to requirements in 29 CFR 1910.1030, used to indicate the presence of a biohazard.

**urethral stricture**—lesion that reduces the inside diameter of the urethra, typically caused by inflammation.

**vector-borne transmission**—transmission of a disease-causing organism through an outside source, or vector.

**virulence**—degree of pathogenicity of a microorganism.

**virus**—microorganism that resides within other living cells and cannot reproduce outside a living cell.

**waterborne**—microorganism carried or transmitted by water.

**willful violation**—a violation of an OSHA standard that an employer knowingly commits or commits with indifference to the law. The penalty for each violation is $5000 to $70,000.

**window phase**—time of exposure to a disease until a serum test reads "positive."

# Index

NOTE: Page numbers in **bold type** refer to information contained in figures.

Antiviral drugs
    avian influenza and, 136
    chickenpox and, 139
Aphasia
    defined, 194
    rabies and, 168
APIC *See* Association for
    Professionals in Infection
    Control and Epidemiology
Appendix, vermiform, 47, 48–49
Arthritis, septic, 147, 202
Association for Professionals in
    Infection Control and
    Epidemiology (APIC), 25, 194
    safe work practices and, 71
    website, 93
Asymptomatic, defined, 194
Asymptomatic infection
    with hepatitis C (HCV), 87
    with HIV, 132
Attenuated, defined, 194
Attenuated varicella vaccine,
    140–141
Augmentin, pneumonia and, 167
Autoimmune disorders, 50, 58
Autoimmune response, 49–50, 194
Avian (bird) influenza, 36
    overview of, 135–137

B
B cells *See* B lymphocytes
B lymphocytes (B cells), **54**,
    57–58, 195
Bacteremia, systemic, 147, 203
Bacteria, 35, 36
    defined, 35, 195
    endogenous flora, 79
    exogenous flora, 79
    immune response to, 49, 52, 56
    intestinal, 48–49, 52
Bacterial meningitis, 35
Basophils, 57, 195
Bell's palsy
    defined, 195
    Lyme disease and, 158
Biohazard containers, 65–67, **66**
    defined, 195

Biohazards
    labeling and, 67, **68**
    universal biohazard symbol,
        67, **69**
    *see also* Biological agents used
        as weapons
Biological agents used as weapons,
    36, 95–107
    advantages and disadvantages
        of, 98–99
    agents, probable, 102–103
    bioterrorism versus biological
        warfare, 103
    Category A agents, 102
    Category B agents, 103
    Category C agents, 103
    current perspectives and
        resources, 100–102
    delivery devices, probable,
        103–104
    health care provider safety, 105
    history of, 98–99, 100
    prevention and surveillance,
        104–105
    public health systems and,
        104–105
Biological terrorism, defined, 195
    *see also* Biological agents used as
        weapons; Bioterrorism
Biological warfare, 103, 195
Biological weapons, U.S. program
    in, 98, **99**, 100
    *see also* Biological agents used as
        weapons
Bioterrorism
    defined, 102, 103, 195
    versus biological warfare, 103
    *see also* Biological agents used as
        weapons
Bird flu (avian influenza), 36,
    135–137
Blackburn, Luke, 100
Bleach, 85
Blood spills, cleanup, 88
Bloodborne pathogens
    alcohol-based hand cleaners
        and, 65